Promoting Children´s Oral Health

Theory & Practice

Aubrey Sheiham
Marcelo Bönecker

Richard G. Watt
Wagner Marcenes
Cesar Messias de Oliveira
Cecile Soriano Rodrigues
Simone Tetu Moysés
Samuel Jorge Moysés
Sabrina Susan Fuller
Claides Abegg
Maria do Carmo Matias Freire
Valeria Coelho Catão Marinho

Quintessence Editora Ltda.
Chicago, London, Berlin, Tokyo, Barcelona, Beijing, Istanbul, Milan,
Moscow, Mumbai, Paris, Prague, São Paulo, Seoul, Warsaw

quintessence
editora ltda.

Title in portuguese: Promovendo Saúde Bucal na Infância e Adolescência Conhecimentos e Práticas

Title in english: Promoting Children´s Oral Health Theory & Practice

Authors: Aubrey Sheiham
Marcelo Bönecker

Translation: Ananyr Porto Fajardo

Design and Cover: Gilberto R. Salomão

ISBN: 85-87425-60-9

quintessence
editora ltda.

Rua Dr. Cesário Mota Jr., 187 – Vila Buarque
01221-020 – São Paulo – SP – Brasil
Tel.: (55 11) 221-1398 – Fax: (55 11) 221-1932
E-mail: quintedit@aol.com

Authors

Aubrey Sheiham
Professor of Dental Public Health, Dept of Epidemiology and Public Health, University College London – England

Marcelo Bönecker
BDS, MSc, PRD, Post Doctor
Senior Lecturer, Dept. of Paediatric Dentistry, University of Sao Paulo (USP) – SP –Brazil
Honorary Lecturer, Dept. of Paediatric Dentistry, CPO Sao Leopoldo Mandic – Brazil

Richard G. Watt
BDS, MSc, PhD, MFPH
Reader and Specialist in Dental Public Health – University College London – England

Wagner Marcenes
BDS, MSc, PhD
Professor of Oral Epidemiology Center for Oral Biometrics, Dental Institute Barts and The London, QMUL, University of London – England

Cesar Messias de Oliveira
BDS, MSc, PRD, Post Doctor
Honorary Research Assistant, Dept. of Epidemiology and Public Health, University College London (UCL) – England

Cecile Soriano Rodrigues
BDS, PhD
Assistant Professor, Dept of Community Dentistry. University of Pernambuco (UPE) – Brazil

Simone Tetu Moysés
BDS, MSc, PRD
Professor Dept. of Epidemiology and Public Health, Pontifical Catholic University of Parana (PUC) – Brazil

Claides Abegg
BDS, PhD
Assistant Professor, Dept. of Community Dentistry Federal University of Rio Grande do Sul (UFRGS) Brazil

Maria do Carmo Matias Freire
BDS, MSc, PRD
Dept. of Dental Public Health Federal University of Goias (UFG) Brazil

Valéria Coelho Catão Marinho
BDS, MSc, PRD
Lecturer Dept. of Epidemiology and Public Health, University College London (UCL) England

Samuel Jorge Moysés
BDS, MSc, PhD
Professor Dept. of Epidemiology and Public Health, Pontifical Catholic University of Parana (PUC) Brazil
Professor Dept. of Epidemiology and Public Health, Federal University Parana (UFPR) Brazil

Sabrina Susan Fuller
MSc, LDS RCS (Edin), MFPHM
Specialist in Dental Public Health
Senior Dental Officer Tameside and Glossop Primary Care Trust, UK
Honorary Lecturer in Oral Health Promotion, University of Manchester England

Preface

This book is memorable for a number of reasons. It is the first comprehensive book in dentistry on promoting the oral health of younger people. The chapters reflect the philosophy of the 'new public health' in general, and oral health promotion in particular. For me, it is a significant personal milestone as the authors are my past students and colleagues. They have forged a coherent unique approach to oral public health from the ideas they gleaned whilst at University College London. I hope that their ideas will spread so that when we look back we shall see how far the discipline of oral public health has advanced. More importantly, the oral health of the public will be bettered by the application of the concepts outlined in this book.

Professor Aubrey Sheiham

Contents

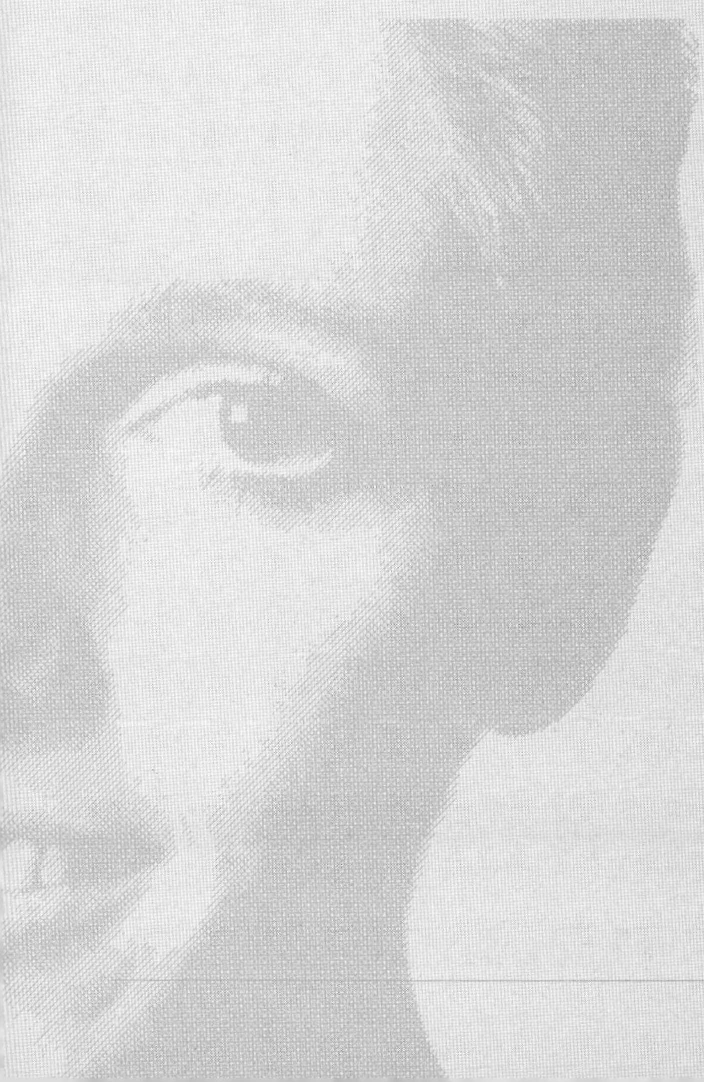

Introduction

Dr. Richard G. Watt

The provision of high quality evidence based treatment and care is the primary function of the dental profession. In addition, dentists and their team members have an important role to play in the prevention of oral diseases and the promotion of oral health. However the prevention of oral diseases has received relatively little attention in terms of resources, research and teaching. The education and payment systems in most parts of the world, including Brasil very much focus on the treatment of dental problems. It is becoming increasingly recognised that treatment services alone will never successfully tackle oral health problems in the population. Even in very rich countries like Sweden with highly developed dental services and large numbers of dental personnel, oral health problems still occur amongst many groups. Dental treatment is not a cure for oral diseases.

Greater recognition is therefore now being placed on exploring ways to effectively promote oral health. Preventive interventions, as with modern treatments need to be developed based upon current scientific knowledge and understanding. This chapter will provide an introduction to a public health approach to prevention for children. The limitations of traditional approaches to prevention will be highlighted and the principles of oral health promotion will be outlined as a more effective means of promoting oral health and reducing inequalities across the child population.

Public health approach to disease prevention

What does a public health approach mean? Most health professionals work at an individual level providing clinical treatment and care to their patients. A minority of doctors, dentists and other health professionals operate at a population level involved in disease monitoring, service planning and community based prevention. All health professionals however need to understand the relevance of a public health perspective in disease prevention. Table 1 lists a set of core public health principles relevant to prevention.

Public health agenda in prevention

- Focuses action on public health problems
- Aims to reduce health inequalities and promote equity
- Addresses the underlying causes of disease in society

- Facilitates self care and independence amongst the population
- Works in partnership with a range of agencies and sectors.
- Utilises an evidence based approach to the design and evaluation of interventions.

Oral diseases are important public health problems in Brasil (Table 2). Although oral health improvements have taken place in recent years, oral diseases are very prevalent and their impact on both society and the individual are significant. Pain, discomfort, sleepless nights and time off school are common problems for many Brazilian children. The costs of treatment are high, although the causes of the diseases are known and are largely preventable. Indeed many middle class Brazilian children now enjoy good oral health. Addressing social inequalities in oral health is a key challenge facing the dental profession.

Criteria for public health problem

- High prevalence of condition
- Impact of condition on individual great (mortality, morbidity, quality of life)
- Impact of condition on wider society (costs of treatment, time off school, lost productivity)
- Condition preventable

The traditional preventive approach

In dentistry, preventive activities have followed a very clinical model. In this approach clinical preventive agents such as topical fluorides and fissure sealants are used in conjunction with chair side educational counselling. This style of approach, often referred to as the "medical model" relies on the expertise and skill of the dentist. The patient is required to comply passively with the dentists' instructions. Regular dental attendance is considered an essential requirement to secure good oral health. The educational component focuses primarily on developing the patients' oral health knowledge based upon the belief that this will lead to changes in the patients' oral hygiene and dietary behaviours. This approach to prevention has been applied to both individual chair side and community, mostly school based programmes and has been the dominant style of preventive action in dentistry. Case study 1 illustrates this approach in more detail.

Case study 1

Dr. John Spencer has worked as a paediatric dentist for the last 20 years. He works part time 3 days a week as a public health dentist for the municipal authority in his city and spends the other 2 days working as a teacher and researcher in the paediatric department of the local dental school.Dr Martins has been interested in preventive dentistry for many years and has established a range of preventive programmes. His particular interest is working with underprivileged children in the large favelas that are located on the edge of his city.His preventive programmes focus on improving the childrens' oral health knowledge, tooth brushing skills and access to services in the local community health centre. Each child in the target area attends at least one dental health education class over a three year period. Over the years he has evaluated a variety of programmes and has demonstrated improvements in the childrens' knowledge 6 weeks after completion of the oral health classes. Recently Dr Martins has become increasingly stressed and depressed about his work. The clinical condition of the children attending the health centre has not improved. He is aware that most children only attend when they have a particular problem. The population in the favela has grown steadily and the demands on the clinic are increasing. Teachers in the local school are no longer interested in the oral health programme due to other demands on their time. Dr Martins now questions whether his work has had any real effect.Discussion points:

- what are the limitations of the preventive approach adopted by Dr Martins?
- how could the preventive programme be improved?

Limitations of conventional dental health education

In recent years, in line with the evidence based movement in clinical medicine the effectiveness of preventive interventions has been scrutinised to determine what interventions are effective and identify those that produce minimal benefit. A whole range of areas of prevention, including smoking, alcohol, injury, nutrition and oral health have been subjected to effectiveness reviews.

How effective have oral health interventions been in improving oral health? Since 1994 a series of different reviews have attempted to answer this question (1-5). Overall very similar methodologies were employed in each review (Table 3).

Effectiveness review methodology

Step 1: Define area of interest – select appropriate key words
Step 2: Systematic search of published and sometimes unpublished literature
Step 3: Define quality assessment criteria (inclusion and exclusion criteria)
Step 4: Assess quality of identified studies – exclude studies who fail defined criteria
Step 5: Summarise overall findings for included studies
Step 6: Present discussion and conclusions

Although the basic steps in conducting an effectiveness review are standard, the findings across the different reviews are not entirely the same. The principal reason for this variation in results is the different quality assessment criteria that have been developed to assess the identified studies. Overall, however, certain consistent results were identified by the reviewers (6) (Table 4).

Common findings of effectiveness reviews

- Many studies were poorly designed and lacked detailed evaluation
- Water fluoridation is effective at preventing dental caries. Fluoride toothpaste is another effective method of delivering fluoride.
- Improving individuals' knowledge of oral health can be achieved in the short term but the effects on behaviour and clinical outcomes are very limited
- Provision of health information alone does not produce long term behaviour changes
- Interventions at an individual level are effective at reducing plaque levels only in the short term
- School based toothbrushing campaigns aimed at improving oral hygiene are largely ineffective
- Mass media campaigns are ineffective at promoting either knowledge or behaviour change

- Very few studies have assessed the effects of interventions on sugars consumption at an individual or population level

Publication of these reviews caused a good deal of debate and discussion within the international dental public health community. Some people concluded that the disappointing results indicated that oral health interventions were ineffective and a waste of resources. Others took a more constructive approach and identified that the majority of the interventions reviewed were in fact educational in nature and that other types of approaches needed to be implemented and fully evaluated.

The findings and conclusions of the oral health effectiveness reviews are very much consistent with the results of reviews in other areas of prevention. A powerful body of international evidence demonstrates the need for a radically different approach to disease prevention. Educational approaches alone have limited effects and may in fact increase inequalities (7). The World Health Organisation and a range of government expert reports have identified a new way forward to promote health and well being. It is essential that those working in dentistry are not left behind but become actively involved in a range of exciting and innovative developments.

Principles of oral health promotion

The modern health promotion movement emerged out of the need for a fundamental change in strategy to improve health and reduce inequalities. Recognition and frustration with the limited value health education interventions could achieve in isolation, led to a rediscovery of a public health approach to prevention. The upstream-downstream allegory illustrates this point very clearly[8] (Figure 1).

Upstream-downstream

A woman was standing by the side of a river enjoying the fine view when she heard a cry of a drowning person. Immediately she jumped in to rescue him, pulled him to the bank and applied artificial respiration. Just as the rescued man was recovering there were more cries from other drowning people in the river. In jumped the rescuer, brought more back and resuscitated them one by one. Exhausted by the numerous cries for help, she then enlisted the help of some helpers and resuscitation equipment. Still she could not cope with the increasing numbers of people in need. The teams worked faster and brought more advanced equipment. However the numbers of drowning people became so numerous that some could not be saved. How could she stop them drowning? Someone suggested swimming lessons were the solution. Midstream swimming lessons were then organised for those in the water. Different educational techniques were used but still more and more people kept flowing down the river crying for help. These rescuing and training activities kept everyone so busy that at no time did anyone stop to consider why people who could not swim were in the river in the first place. Who or what was pushing them in upstream?
Discussion point:

- What factors 'upstream' create poor oral health?
- Outline actions that could be implemented 'upstream' to promote and maintain oral health?

The dental profession have largely concentrated their efforts on 'downstream' action when the damage has already been done. Certain motivated members of the profession have ventured up to the mid-

Fig. 1 Upstream-downstream.

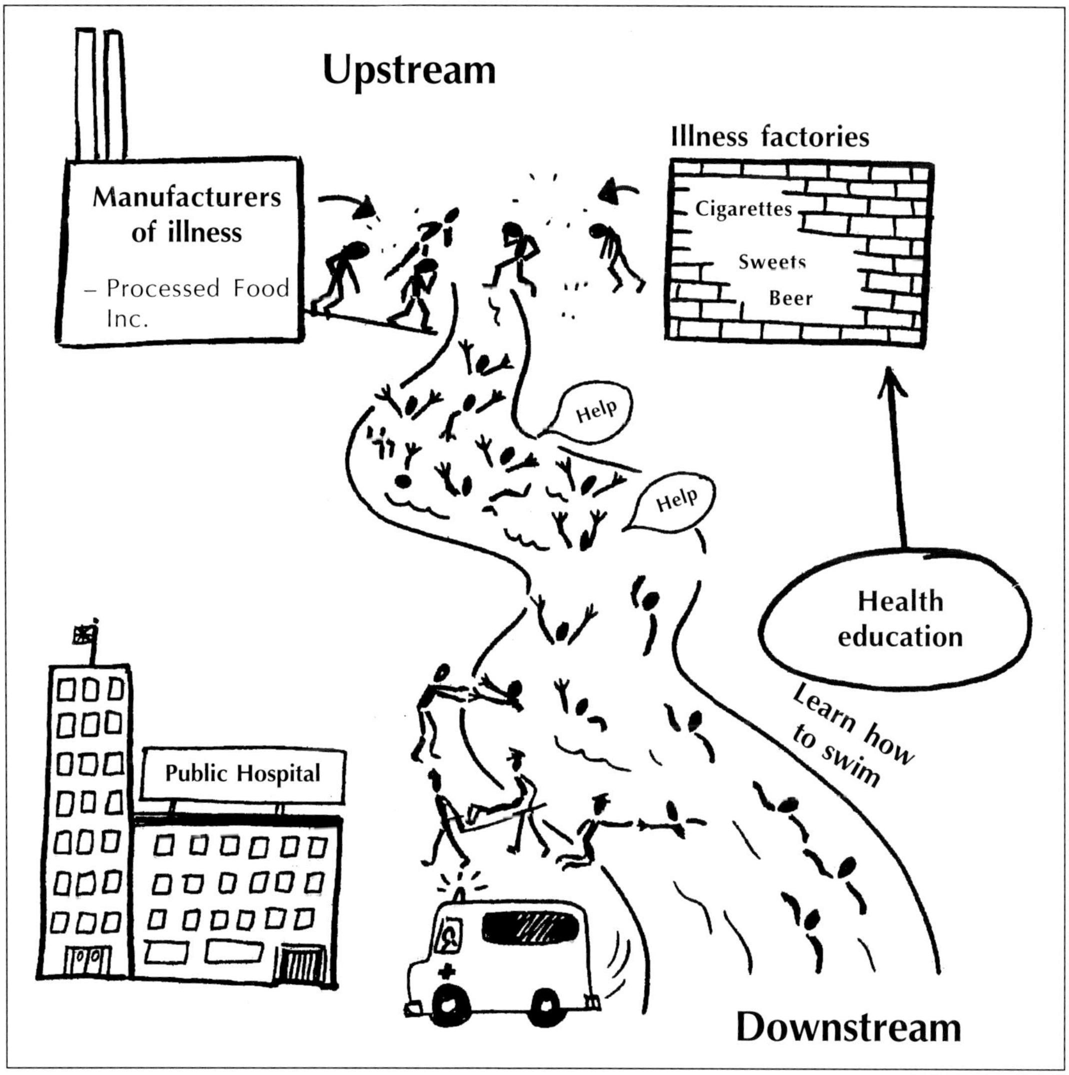

stream and have focused their efforts on developing educational action to promote better oral health. What about 'upstream' action? Instead of concentrating so much time and effort on 'downstream and mid-stream' activities, more effort should be directed at making the "river shallower" – making the healthier choices the easier choices[9].

Many definitions of health promotion have been proposed but the World Health Organisation definition has been widely adopted as a useful description of contemporary practice:

"Health promotion is the process of enabling individuals and communities to increase control over the determinants of health and thereby improve their health. Health promotion represents a mediating strategy between people and their environment, combining personal choice and social responsibility for health to create a healthier future."[10]

The essence of contemporary health promotion practice is the need to address the underlying causes of ill health in society, the determinants of health.

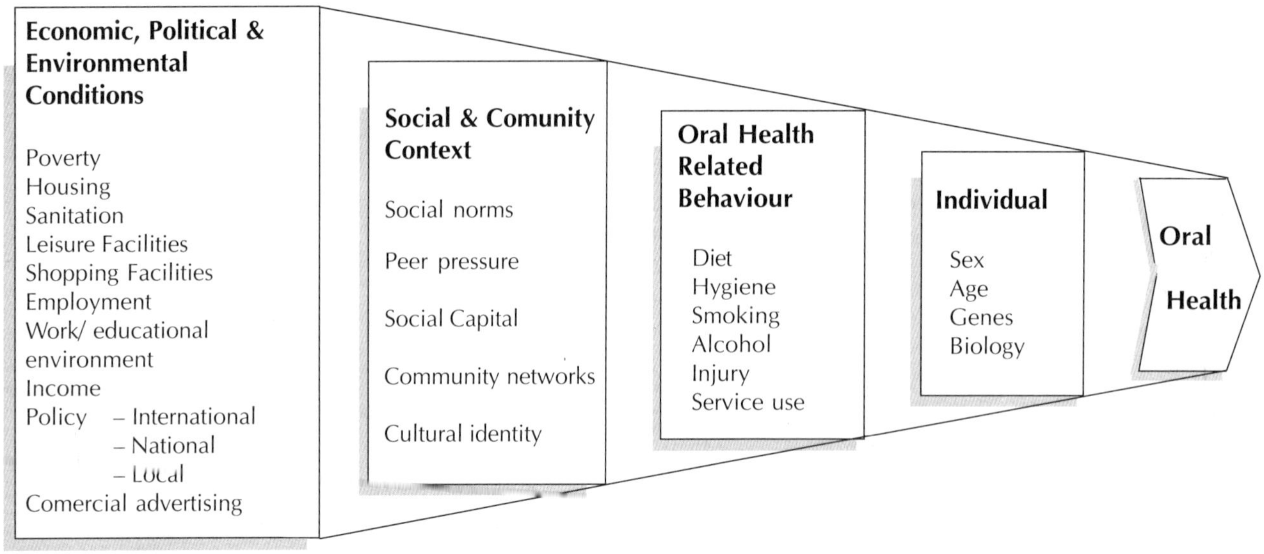

Fig. 2 – Social determinants of oral health.

Social determinants of disease

What are the causes of dental diseases? Traditionally dental health education interventions have sought to alter behaviours and lifestyles which are seen to be the cause of dental problems. Programmes therefore focus on oral hygiene skills, changing inappropriate dietary patterns and encouraging frequent dental attendance. However this narrow and very often 'victim blaming' approach fails to recognise the mounting evidence highlighting the importance of, what is termed the social determinants of health. Public health research and policy development now recognise the underlying importance on health and disease of economic, political, environmental and social factors.[11,12] Social conditions and structure are the true aetiological agents in most chronic diseases[13] Health promotion is directed at the underlying determinants, the causes of the causes.

Figure 2 presents an overview of the social determinants of oral health. The essence of this model is the recognition of the impact of the broader social environment on lifestyle behaviours. Oral health related behaviours are not just simple actions but are enmeshed in more complex socio-environmental conditions (14). For example, how much sugar an adolescent eats is determined by a complex range of interconnecting factors, the behaviour is in essence merely an expression of these underlying factors. Dietary patterns are influenced by a range of social factors. At an immediate level, family and friends influence what a teenager will eat. Changing social trends in eating and cultural norms also have a powerful effect. At the macro level economic, environmental and political factors have an overriding impact on nutritional patterns. Cost, access, transport, policy, advertising and the availability of choices all determine what is eaten. Indeed this approach to understanding the causes of oral diseases also applies to many other chronic conditions and is the basis for joint working across agencies and sectors.

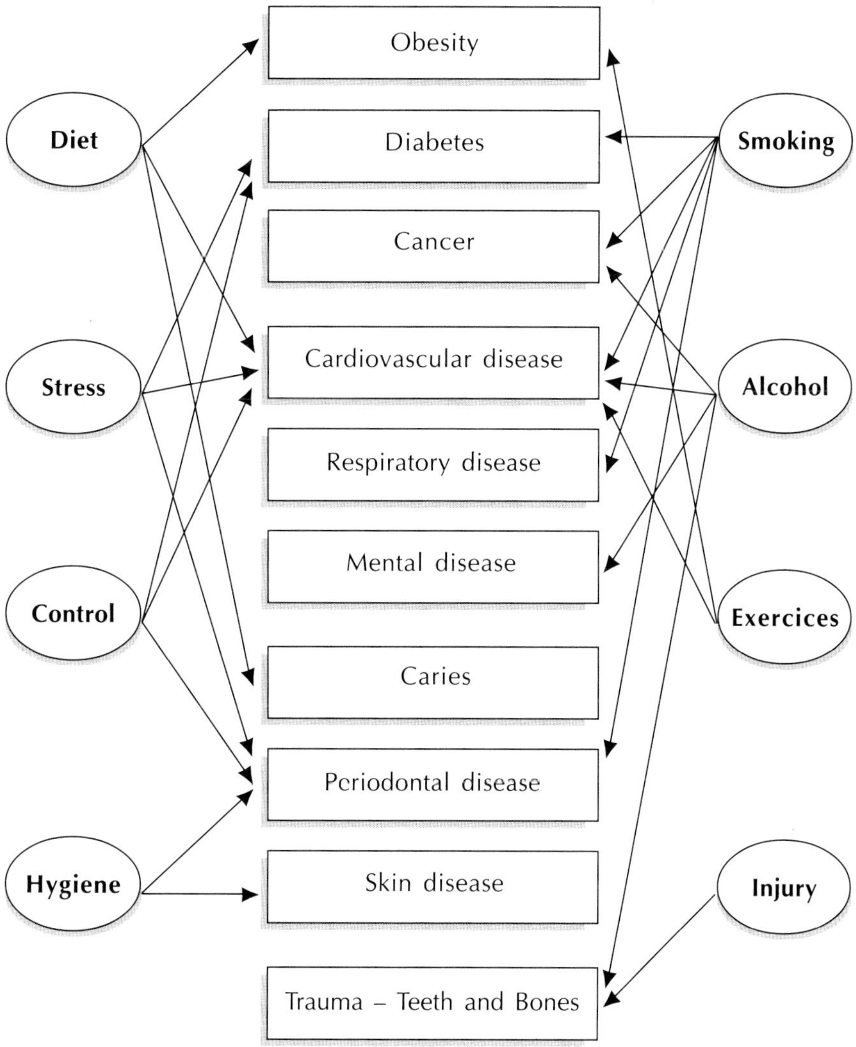

Fig. 3 Common risk factor approach.

Social determinants of oral health

Common risk factor approach

One of the major criticisms of traditional dental health education has been it's narrow, isolated and compartmentalised approach, essentially separating the mouth from the rest of the body. All too often programmes have been developed in isolation from other health initiatives. This uncoordinated approach can at best lead to a duplication of effort but often in fact results in conflicting and contradictory messages being delivered to the public. The common risk factor approach recognises that the chronic conditions which are the major public health problems across the globe such as heart disease, stroke, cancers, diabetes, mental illness and oral diseases share a set of common risks (Figure 3). An inadequate diet, smoking, poor hygiene, stress and trauma are factors linked to the development of several chronic conditions including oral diseases (15). The key concept of the integrated common risk approach is that by directing action on these common risks and their underlying social determinants, improvements in a range of chronic conditions will be achieved more efficiently and with greater effectiveness (13). The common risk factor approach provides a rational for joined up working, a key principle of health promotion practice.

Partnership working

Many dentists may feel very uncertain and anxious how they can become involved in health promotion practice which seems so far removed from clinical dentistry. How can dentists change the living conditions of the most vulnerable children in society? How can clinicians take on the power of multi-national companies? The answer to these questions is quite simply that dentists alone cannot expect to achieve meaningful results. However when effective partnerships are formed with a range of relevant and influential groups then results can indeed be achieved. The challenge is to place oral health issues onto the broader agenda. A collection of different partners have a direct influence on oral health (Table 5).

Potential partners in oral health promotion

- Other health professionals: doctors, pharmacists, nurses, community health workers.
- Education services: head teachers, education planners, teachers, support staff.
- Local government services: planning departments, social workers, catering services, local politicians.
- Voluntary sector: community groups, religious groups.
- Industry and commerce: food retailers, advertisers, water industry, drug companies.
- National government: education department, agriculture, trade.

Traditionally dentists have been trained in isolation from other health professionals. The knowledge and skills required to work in a collaborative manner are not covered in most under graduate dental curriculae. How can this style of working be facilitated? Partnership working needs to satisfy three basic points:

1. Demonstrating relevance and importance
2. Acknowledging common agendas for change and shared goals
3. Offering unique expertise, contacts and skills

Oral diseases are rarely fatal conditions and to many may seem rather unimportant and peripheral. Socio-dental research has however highlighted the wide range of impacts oral conditions can have on both individual quality of life and at a societal level. For example, pain, discomfort, sleepless nights and time off school are all effects of oral diseases on children's quality of life. Lost productivity due to time off work attending dental services and economic costs to the health services of providing dental services are examples of society wide impacts. Many groups in society can be persuaded of the importance of oral health when meaningful and relevant impacts are demonstrated.

As outlined above the common risk factor approach provides a rational agenda for setting shared goals with other sectors and agencies. For example, diets high in sugar are not only linked to the development of dental caries but also have an effect on obesity and nutrient depletion. The World Health Organisation has recommended that sugars should be reduced to a maximum of 10% of energy intake or 60 g/day/person (16). Essentially oral health should be considered an integral part of general health and action focused on common risks and conditions.

What expertise and skills can dentists offer other groups? This clearly depends on many diverse factors but often public health dentists may already have established good working relationships with sectors such as the local education service. Oral health epidemiological data on children is often more readily available than other forms of health data. As a consequence oral health population based data can be used as an indicator of general health status and as a marker for health inequalities. Another potential unique feature is the fact that unlike most other health services, young people often attend dental services on a regular basis. This provides an opportunity of working with young people directly and assessing more clearly their needs and concerns.

From prescription to participation

Rather than adopting the conventional 'top down' approach in which professionals control decisions and dictate action to the community, effective health promotion requires professionals to work with members of the community in a participative manner. A 'bottom up' approach aims to share control and facilitate joint decision making. This approach respects the expertise and knowledge non professionals have and aims to harness collective skills for the benefit of promoting better health and achieving sustainable improvements.

Working with the community takes time, resources and appropriate skills. In addition identifying relevant and appropriate community representatives requires knowledge of the local community groups and organisations. In parts of Brasil community representation and involvement in social and health policy has developed much further than in many other parts of the world. This provides a valuable resource in health promotion action.

Complementary actions to improve oral health

A key finding from the oral health promotion effectiveness reviews was recognition of the limitations of health education as the sole means of promoting oral health and reducing inequalities. Increasing individual's knowledge is one element of improving oral health. However a change in knowledge does not lead automatically to any sustained alteration in behaviour. Indeed improved oral health knowledge may be of limited value for those who live in an environment where positive oral health choices are not available. In these circumstances other strategies will be required. A shift in emphasis is needed away from a sole reliance on educational actions to one in which a range of complementary strategies can be implemented appropriate to the needs and circumstances of the target population.

The first international health promotion conference in Ottawa, Canada held in 1984 published a set of guiding principles for effective action. The Ottawa Charter, although over 16 years old, still provides a radical agenda for change and is frequently used as a framework to guide good practice (10). In many countries dental professionals are using these principles to inform the development of oral health strategies.

The Ottawa Charter outlines five key areas of health promotion action:

1. Promoting health through public policy: by focusing attention on health of public policies from all sectors, and not just the health sector.
2. Creating supportive environments: by assessing the impact of the environment and clarifying opportunities to make changes conducive to health.
3. Developing personal skills: by moving beyond the transmission of information, to promote understanding, and to support the development of per-

analyzed. This means that if a child who shows a DMF-S = 7 for having 7 surfaces with caries lesion will continue with the same DMF-S = 7 all their lives even though the lesions have been treated and filled, since the 7 "D" units will become 7 "F" units. Moreover, this value of DMF-S = 7 for this child will be the same or higher during his or her whole life and never decrease. In face of these shortcomings, two indexes were developed that overcome the problems of the DMF/dmf indexes.

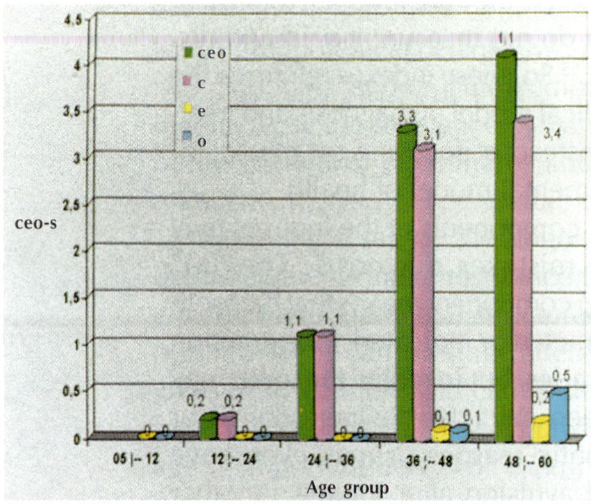

Figure 1.1 Distribution of the mean dmf-s index according to the age group, in months. Diadema, São Paulo, 1997.

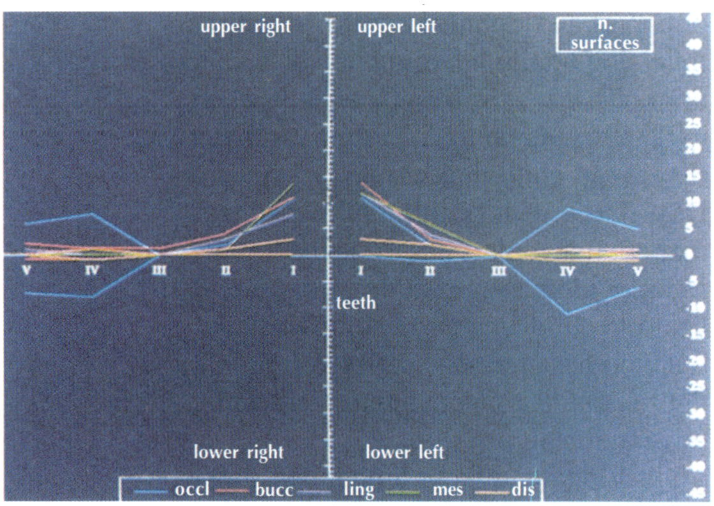

Figure 1.2 Distribution of the number of caries lesions, by dental arch, tooth, and surface in 2 years old children. Diadema, São Paulo, 1997.

The Index of Functional Teeth (IFT) is based on the principle that filled teeth (F component) are functional. So it proposes adding filled teeth or surfaces to the sound ones. These two components of the index receive identical weight based on the fact that they play equivalent functions in the clinical condition. In this way, it reflects the influence of the restorative approach on oral health, which is considered prevention at a secondary level.[66] This index, in a general way, has a stronger emphasis on health (addition of healthy components) and not on disease (addition of decayed, missing, and filled).

The Healthy Teeth Equivalent Index, known as T- Health (Healthy Tissue), aims to report the amount of healthy tissue possessed by a person at a given time. A sound tooth, for example, has more healthy tissue than a filled tooth that, in turn has more healthy tissue than a tooth with a caries lesion. Based on this reasoning, the tooth indicated for extraction does not have any healthy tissue. In order to obtain numerical results for the index, sound, filled, and carious teeth received scores 4, 2, and 1, respectively. A Brazilian study,[67] however, showed that, in reality, filled and carious teeth have approximately the same amount of healthy tissue. So, T-Health can be used with the score 1 for filled teeth.

There are other indexes and methodologies for examination which also aim to simplify the DMF/dmf index and to optimize their interpretation.[68] An alternative is to by-pass the limitations of the DMF/dmf indexes, in relation to the fact that their components have identical weight. One can analyze the composition of theses indexes considering the individual contributions of each of their components. The sum of the mean value of each of the components (D, M, F / d, m, f) must be equal to the mean value of the total DMF/dmf. In this way, the analysis indicates, for example, if the component decayed or filled was the one that had the higher impact on the index's composition. This information is of great importance for planning and executing dental services[69] (Fig. 1.1).

Besides knowing which component contributes the most to the index, it becomes important to know on which teeth and/or surfaces it was more prevalent, since indexes do not have this information. In general, when the index's value is low, the majority of the caries lesions occur on occlusal surfaces and fissures. When the index's value increases, more free and approximal surfaces are attacked[69] (Figs. 1.2, 1.3 and 1.4).

The significance of knowing the hierarchy in the distribution of caries is based on the fact that, if the majority of the lesions were occlusal, it would only be necessary occlusal fillings or sealants. This fact determines the type of personnel and essential training to deal with the population's treatment needs. Moreover, the distribution helps in planning preventive strategies, since as the caries prevalence decreases, a decrease in the caries prevalence located on less susceptible sites (approximal and free surfaces) occurs. They are more difficult and expensive to treat. Most of the caries will be on more susceptible sites (occlusal pit and fissure surfaces of first molars).[69,70]

Besides the indexes described, the need to know the subjectively perceived health condition, or the impact of oral health conditions on the quality of life, has lead to the development of sociodental indicators.[68,71,72] Such indicators, can complement the traditional indicators. What they aim to do is reveal perceived impacts of oral health problems on the quality of life of people. One, the Child-OIDP, has been designed specifically for use with children.[73]

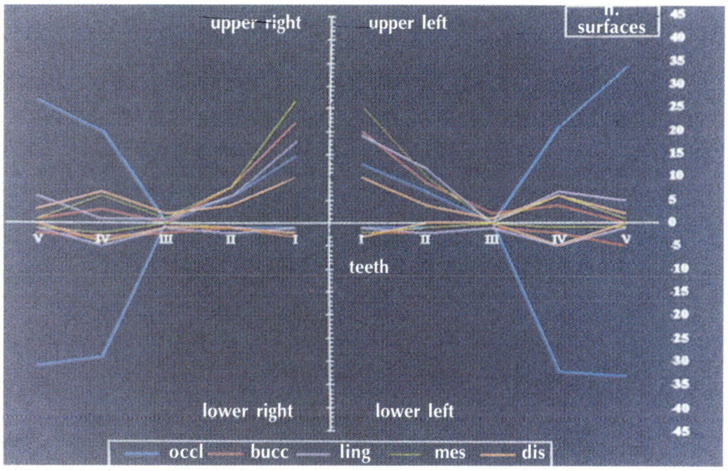

Figure 1.3 Distribution caries lesions by dental arch, tooth, and surface, in 3 year-old children. Diadema, São Paulo, 1997.

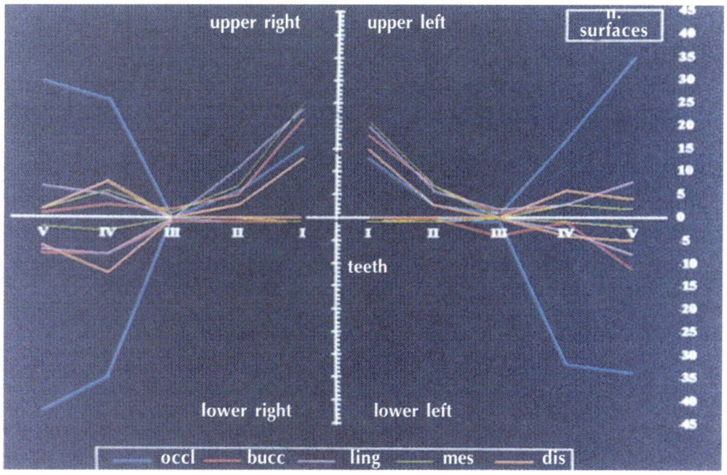

Figure 1.4 Distribution of the number of caries lesions by dental arch, tooth, and surface in 4 year-old children. Diadema, São Paulo, 1997.

Caries experience in children. The case of Brazil

In many respects the patterns and trends in caries in Brazil are illustrative of patterns of caries in children.

Caries experience in deciduous teeth

There are few studies on babies and pre-school children. [69,74-89] The percentage of children with caries lesion varies, for example, from 0 to 23% in 1 year-old children; 13 to 69% in 3 years old children; and 35 to 56% in 5 years old children. The trends in caries prevalence in children from 5 to 59 months of age has been observed and reported since 1995 until recently in the city of Diadema, near São Paulo[89]. The four cross-sectional studies done with the same protocol in 1995, 1997, 1999 and 2002 show a significant decline in both prevalence and severity of caries. For example, the prevalence of

Box 1.1 dmf-t index of the main national epidemiologic studies performed in the last 20 years, according to age group.

Author	Year	City	dmf-t				
			0–12	12–24	24–36	36–48	48–60
Detogni	1994	Xingu	–	–	2.33	8.50	8.35
Pinto	1996	Nacional	–	–	–	1.76	2.57
Carvalho	1996	Brasília**	–	0.36	1.50	2.13	2.78
Freire	1996	Goiânia	–	0.09	0.40	1.14	2.18
Bönecker	1997	Diadema	0	0.23	1.33	–	–
Assis	1997	Guarulhos*	0.07	0.75	1.32	–	–
Cerqueira	1998	Natal	0	0.32	2.31	–	–
Dini	1998	Araraquara*	–	–	–	–	1.18
Bönecker	2000	Diadema	0	0.11	0.65	1.79	2.19
Bönecker	2000	Diadema**	0	0.23	1.16	2.29	2.51

Source: bibliographic references.
* Considers age groups jointly.
** Considers incipient lesions.

caries in 2 to 3 year-old children was 45%, 29%, and 18% in 1995, 1997, and 1999, respectively. However, children who belonged to the same birth cohort showed an increase in the prevalence of caries, measured by the dmf index. Children under 1 years old had on average,a dmf-s 0.0 in 1995; two years later, in 1997, this population group had a dmf-s 1.1, and two years later, in 1999, this same population group of children now aged 4 years old had a dmf-s 3.2 (Fig. 1.5).

The direct comparison between Brazilian and international studies is difficult due to methodological questions. In general, the caries experience in Brazilian babies and preschool children is a slightly higher than elsewhere.[90-98]

Box 1.2 dmf-s index of the main national epidemiologic studies performed in the last 20 years, by age group.

Author	Year	City	dmf-t				
			0–12	12–24	24–36	36–48	48–60
Mattos-Graner	1994	Piracicaba*	–	–	1.41	–	–
Tomita	1994	Bauru*	–	–	1.18	–	–
Tomita	1994	São Paulo*	–	–	0.43	–	–
Carvalho	1996	Brasília**	–	0.68	2.06	4.10	5.42
Bönecker	1997	Diadema	0	0.43	1.99	–	–
Assis	1997	Guarulhos*	0.07	0.90	1.46	–	–
Cerqueira	1997	Natal	0	0.34	3.35	–	–
Bönecker	2000	Diadema	0	0.21	1.09	3.34	4.09
Bönecker	2000	Diadema**	0	0.34	1.75	4.05	4.50
Bönecker	2002	Diadema	0	0.21	1.02	2.32	3.19

Source: bibliographic references.
* Considers age groups jointly.
** Considers incipient lesions.

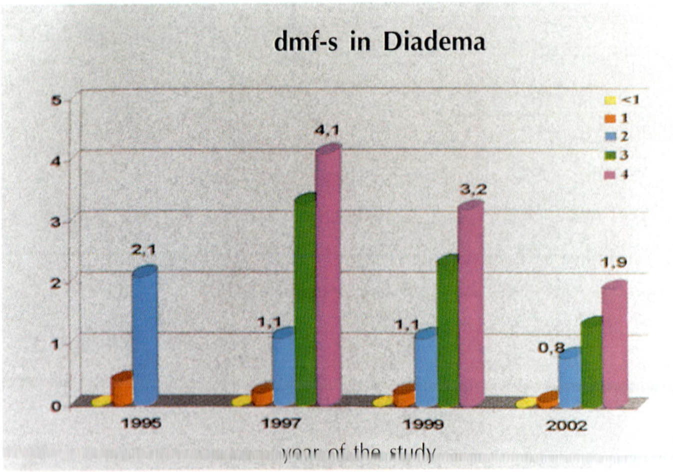

Figure 1.5 Mean dmf-s index by age group and year of study. Diadema, São Paulo, 1995, 1997, 1999, and 2000.

Box 1.3 DMF-T index of the main national epidemiologic studies performed in Brazilian municipalities where surveys were done twice or more.

Author	City	Year	DMFT	Year	DMFT
Dini	Araraquara	1989	3.40	1992	2.80
M. Saúde	Bacabal	1976	6.88	1987	2.68
Viegas	Barretos	1971	8.37	1987	3.54
Prefeitura	Blumenau	1968	8.00	1998	1.39
Viegas	Campinas	1961	7.36	1976	3.30
Prefeitura	Curitiba	1981	10.1	1997	1.81
Prefeitura	Diadema	1995	2.37	1997	1.81
Marcenes	Florianópolis	1971	9.17	1997	3.00
Ogawa	Londrina	1981	6.95	1992	3.39
Moreira	Paulínia	1980	8.20	1994	3.00
Kalamatianos	S. J. Campos	1979	8.05	1986	6.04
Acieri	Uberlândia	1972	11.48	1983	5.50

Caries experience in permanent teeth

There has been a significant improvement in caries experience in permanent teeth of children in industrialized countries and in Brazilian children's.[61,99] The mean caries experience for Brazilian 12 year-old children in 1986 was 6.7, while in 1996 it was 3.1. There were some inconsistencies in the methodology in the two surveys.[100] There is a downward trend in caries prevalence among school children in Brazil.[101-113] A recent systematic review about the tendency of dental caries in 6 and 12 years old children from Latin America and the Caribbean[114] indicates that a decrease in the prevalence of caries occurred between 1970 and 2000 not only in Brazil. The large decreases in caries levels over a 16-year period show that caries levels can be decreased by public health measures. For example, Curitiba had a significant decrease in the caries prevalence for 12 year-old children; from 10.1 to 1.8 between 1981 and 1997 (Box 1.3).

The comparison of caries prevalence in schoolchildren from Brazil with schoolchildren from other countries can be also evaluated through the World Health Organization's data bank. WHO has been collecting caries prevalence data for 12 year-old children from different countries and continents. The Global Oral Health Data Bank,[115] which can be easily accessed by Internet. It is worthwhile highlighting that, while Brazil had a DMF-T 3.1 in 1996 for 12 years old school children, England, Denmark, Finland, and Australia, among many other countries, had a DMF-T around 1.1 at the beginning of the 1990's.

Factors that contributed to the decrease of caries

Factors that may have contributed to the decrease of caries experience in Brazil and in the world have been identified. The majority of the researchers believe that most important factor in the decrease of caries was fluoridated dental toothpaste.[116] Educative and preventive programs for the population have also been considered as factors contributing to the decrease,[117] though this fact has been challenged. Educative and preventive programs had a low impact on the reduction of caries.[118] Other factors that may have contributed to the decrease of caries are the change on the criterion of caries diagnosis,[119] the decrease in sugar intake;[117,120] the use of antibiotics;[121] and the improvement of socioeconomic conditions.[60,122-124]

In Brazil, the decrease of the sugar intake, the change of the philosophy of treatment and the improvement of socioeconomic conditions, as well as water fluoridation, and the access to fluoridated dental toothpastes, are all measures within the context of oral health promotion. They should be emphasized to achieve bigger decreases in the levels of prevalence and severity of dental caries in children and adolescents.

Control of the prevalence and incidence of dental caries

The control of prevalence and incidence of dental caries may be done by the use of two associated strategies. The first is the rational use of fluoride. The second is the decrease in sugar intake and the better oral cleanliness to decrease the dental biofilm.

It seems that the caries disease is very easy to control. However, the idea that health can be controlled by the individual and in this way, improved by simple educational techniques and individual interventions is one of the marks of the medical/biological model to treat and prevent disease,[125] that has been already widely questioned and considered to be of limited effectiveness.[126]

The adoption of a preventive approach to reduce levels of disease by the individual action of health professionals in clinics is very limited. This approach adopts an authoritarian style of action, in which health providers act as specialists for patients who passively receive preventive care. On one hand, children receive personal hygiene and instruction at school on how and what to eat, while on the other hand it is expected that mothers control their children's bad habits at home.[127] In this scenario, what seams to be clear is that a change of approach is needed. One that is more effective and based on evidence-based dental care.

The new approach based on health promotion, as described in the Ottawa Charter[1] for the health promotion in 1987, directs attention to the interaction between people and their environments (psychological, social, cultural, political, economic, biologic, and environmental). This approach is based on new public health policies and the creation of healthy environments that makes healthy choices the easier choices. These strategies and many others will be elaborated in Chapters 5 to 10 on health promotion.

In the Oral Health Promotion approaches outlined in this book dental caries control is not limited to the monitoring of its determinant factors (sugars, bacterial biofilms, and fluoride) at an individual level in dental offices. Society needs to be healthy as a whole. Dentists should be advocates for oral health and help offer all people the possibility of living without oral diseases and impairements. They should be on tap, not on top.

Conclusions

In spite of the remarkable worldwide decline in the prevalence of dental caries, caries still is considered an important public health problem. The determinant factors directly related to dental caries are widely known. Caries can be avoided or controlled by the adoption of strategies based on health promotion principles. That approach uses the common risk factor approach (CRFA) and should be adopted in the prevention of dental caries. By using the common risk factor approach dental strategies become an integrated and integral part of strategies for general health promotion elaborated to avoid other chronic diseases.

References

1. OMS: Ottawa Charter for Health Promotion. Health Promotion, 1987; 1 (44).
2. Burt BA, Eklund AS. Dental Caries. In: Burt BA e col. *Dentistry, dental practice and the Community*: Saunders Company, Philadelphia, 1992. 4. ed. p.90-112.
3. Sreebny LM. Sugar availability, sugar consumption and dental caries. *Community Dent Oral Epidemiol,* 1982a;10:1-7.
4. Sreebny LM. The sugar-caries axis. *Int Dent J,* 1982b;32:1-12.
5. Sreebny LM. Cereal availability and dental caries. *Community Dent Oral Epidemiol,* 1983;11:148-155.
6. Takeuchi M. Epidemiological study on dental caries in Japanese children before, during and after World War II. *Int Dent J,* 1961;11:443-57.
7. Toverid G. The influence of war and post-war conditions on the teeth of Norwegian school children. I. Eruption of permanent teeth and status of deciduous dentition. *Milbank Mem Fund Quart,* 1956;34:354-430.
8. Zitzow RE. The relationship of diet and dental caries in the Alaskan eskimo population. *Alaska Med,* 1979; 21:10-14.
9. Möller IJ, Poulsen S, Nielsen V. The prevalence of dental caries in Godhavn and Scoresbysund districts, Greenland. *Scand J Dent Res,* 1972;80:168-180.
10. Holloway PJ, James PMC, Slack GL. Dental disease in Tristan da Cunha. *Br Dent J,* 1963;19-25.
11. Roberts JF, Roberts GJ. Relation between medicines sweetened with sucrose and dental issue. *Br Med J,* 1979;14-16.
12. Gustaffson BE, Quensel CE, Lanke LS, Lunquist C, Grahnen H, Bonow BE, Krasse B. The Vipeholm dental caries study. The effect of different levels of carbohydrate intake on caries activity in 436 individuals observed for five years. *Acta Odontol Scand,* 1954;11:232-264.
13. Harris R. Biology of the children of Hopewood House, Bowral, Australia. Observations on dental caries experience extending over 5 years (1957-61). *J Dent Res,* 1963; 42: 1387-1399.
14. Rodrigues C, Sheiham A. Relationship between dietary guidelines, sugar intake and caries in primary teeth in low income Brazilian 3 years old: a longitudinal study. *Int J Paed Dent,* 2000;10:47-55.
15. Freire MC. Dieta, Saúde Bucal e Saúde Geral. *In*: Buischi Y, *Promoção de saúde bucal na clínica odontológica.* São Paulo: Artes Médicas, 2000; 249-78.
16. Rugg-Gunn AJ, Edgar WM. Sugar and dental caries: a review of the evidence. *Community Dent Health,* 1984;1:85-92.
17. Rugg-Gunn AJ. Nutrition and dental health. Oxford University Press, Oxford. 1993.
18. Freire MCM. Substitutos do açúcar: sua importância na prevenção da cárie. *Rev Bras Odontol,* 1994; 51:38-47.
19. Ripa LW. Nursing caries: a comprehensive review. *Pediatr Dent,* 1988; 10:268-82.
20. Broderick E, Mabry J, Robertson D, Thompson J. Baby bottle tooth decay in native American children in Head Start centers. *Public Health Rep,* 1989; 104:50-54.
21. Tinanoff N, O'Sullivan D. Early childhood caries: overview and recent findings. *Pediatr Dent,* 1997;19:12-16.
22. van Houte P. Role of microorganisms in caries etiology. *J Dent Res,* 1994;73:672-81.
23. van Palenstein Helderman WH, Mattee MIN, van der Hoeven JS, Mikx FH. Cariogenicity depends more on diet than the prevailing mutans streptococcal species. *J Dent Res,* 1995;75:535-45.
24. Krasse B. The effect of caries inducing streptococci in hamsters fed diets with sucrose or glucose. *Arch Oral Biol,* 1965; 10: 223-6.
25. Larson RH, Fitzgerald RJ. Caries development

in rats of differing ages with controlled flora. *Arch Oral Biol,* 1964; 9:663-8.

26. Gibbons RJ, Berman KS. Dental caries and alveolar bone loss in rats infected with capsule forming streptococci of human origin. *Arch Oral Biol,* 1966;11:549-60.
27. Milnes AR, Bowden GHW. The microflora associated with developing lesions of nursing caries. *Carics Res,* 1985;19:289-97.
28. Loesche WJ, Rowan J, Straffon LH, Loos PJ. Association of Streptococcus mutans with human dental decay. *Infect Immun,* 1975; 11:1252-60.
29. Duchen S, van Houte J. Colonization of teeth in human by Streptococcus mutans as related to its concentration in saliva and host age. *Infect Immun,* 1978; 20:120-5.
30. Bercowitz RJ, Turner J, Hughes C. Microbial characteristics of the human dental caries associated with prolonged bottle-feeding. *Arch Oral Biol,* 1984;29:949-91.
31. Van Houte J, Gibbs G, Butera C. Oral flora of children with nursing bottle caries. *J Dent Res,* 1982;61:382-5.
32. Brown JP, Junner C, Liew V. A study of S mutans levels in both infants with bottle caries and their mothers. *Aust Dent J,* 1985;30:96-8.
33. Boue D, Arman E, Turby G. A bacteriological study of rampant caries in children. *J Dent Res,* 1987;66:23-8.
34. Mattee MIN, Mikx FHM, Masille SYM, van Palenstein Helderman WH. Mutans streptococci and lactobacilli in breast fed children with rampant caries. *Caries Res,* 1992;26:183-7.
35. Fujiwara T, Sasada E, Mina N, Ooshima T. Caries prevalence and salivary mutans strptococci in 0-2 year old children of Japan. *Community Dent Oral Epidemiol,* 1991;19:151-4.
36. Alallusua S, Matto J, Gronroos L. Oral colonization by more than one type of mutans streptococci in children with nursing bottle dental caries. *Arch Oral Biol,* 1996;41:167-73.
37. Edelstein B, Tinanoff N. Correlation of dental caries in young children with a non laboratory method of salivary S. mutans sampling. *Pediatric Dent,* 1989;11:129-32.
38. Bretz WA, Djahjah C, Almeida RS, Loesche WJ. Relationship of microbioal and salivary parameters with dental caries in Brazilian pre-school children. Community *Dent Oral Epidemiol,* 1992;20:261-4.
39. Thibodeau EA, O'Sullivan DM, Tinanoff N. Mutans streptococci and caries prevalence in pre-school children. *Communtiy Dent Oral Epidemiol,* 1993; 21: 288-91.
40. Thibodeau EA, O'Sullivan DM. Salivary mutans streptococci and incidence of caries in preschool children. *Caries Res,* 1995; 29:148-53.
41. Berkowitz RJ, Jordan HV, White G. The early establishment of S. mutans in the mouth of infants. *Arch Oral Biol,* 1975;20:171-4.
42. Grindefjord M, Dahlof G, Nelsson B, Moodeer T. Prediction of dental caries development in 1 year-old children. *Caries Res,* 1995;29:343-8.
43. Caufield PW, Cutter GR, Dasanayake AP. Initial acquisition of MS by infants: evidence for a discrete window of infectivity. *J Dent Res,* 1993;72:37-45.
44. Kohler B, Andreen I, Jonsson B. The earlier the colonization by MS, the higher the caries prevalence at 4 years of age. *Oral Microbiol Immunol,* 1988;3:14-17.
45. Roeters FJM, van der Hoeven, JS, Burgesdijk, RC; Schaeken, M.J.M. Lactobacilli, *mutans* streptococi and dental caries: a longitudinl study in 2 years-old children up to the age of 5 years. *Caries Res,* 1995;29:272-9.
46. Grindefjord M, Dahlof G, Nilsson B, Modeer T. Step-wise prediction of dental caries in children up to 3,5 years of age. *Caries Res,* 1996;30:256-66.
47. Seow WK. Biological mechanisms of early childhood caries. *Community Dent Oral Epidemiol,* 1998;26:8-27. Supplement 1.
48. Bönecker M, Ardenghi T, Trindade CP. Transmissão Vertical na infecção por S Mutans. *J Bras Odontoped Odonto Bebê.* Aceito para publicação, 2004.
49. Loesche WJ. Role of *Streptococcus mutans* in dental decay. *Microbiol Rev,* 1986;50: 353-80.
50. van Houte J. Role of microorganisms in caries etiology. *J Dent Res,* 1994;73: 672-81.
51. van Houte J. Bacterial specificity in the etiology of dental caries. *Int Dent J,* 1980; 30:305-26.
52. Klock B, Krasse B. Microbial and salivary conditions in 9-12 years old children. *Scand J Dent Res,* 1977;85:56-63.
53. Mandel ID. The functions of saliva. *J Dent Res,* 1987;66:623-7.
54. Hyypa T, Karhuvaara L, Tenuovo J, Lumikari M, Vilja P. Antimicrobial factors in whole saliva of human infants: a longitudinal study. *Pediatr Dent,* 1989;11:30-6.
55. Tenuovo J, Lagerlöf F. Saliva. *In*: Thylstrup A, Fejerskov O. *Cariologia Clínica.* 2. ed. São Paulo: Ed. Santos; 1995. p.17-43.

56. Carlos JP, Gittelsolm AM. Longitudinal studies of the natural history of caries II. *Arch Oral Biol,* 1965;10:739-51.
57. Seow WK. Enamel hypoplasia in the primary dentition: a review. *J Dent Child,* 1991; 58:441-52.
58. Marcenes W, Bönecker M. Aspectos epidemiológicos e sociais das doenças bucais. *In:* Buischi YP. *Promoção de saúde bucal na clínica odontológica.* São Paulo: Artes Médicas 2000, p.75-98.
59. Black D, Morris JN, Smith C, Townsend P. *The black report.* Ed. Pinguin; 1980.
60. Carmichael CL, Rugg Gunn A, French AD, Cranage JD. The effect of fluoridation upon the relationship between caries experience and social class in 5 year old childrenin Newcastle and Northumberland. *Br Dent J,* 1980;149:163-7.
61. Ministério da Saude. Levantamento epidemiológico em saúde bucal: Brasil, zona urbana, 1986. Divisão Nacional de Saúde Bucal & Fundação Serviços de Saúde Pública. Série C, Estudos e Projetos, 4. Brasília; 1988. 137p.
62. Reisine S, Douglass JM. Psychosocial and behavioural issues in early childhood caries. *Community Dent Oral Epidemiol* 1998;26:supplement 1: 32-44.
63. Klein H, Palmer CE. *Dental caries in American Indian Children.* Public Health Bulletin no. 239. US Government Printing Office.
64. Grubbel AO. A measurement of dental caries prevalence and treatment service for deciduous teeth. *J Dent Res,* 1944; 23: 163-8.
65. Sheiham A, Maizels JE, Cushing AM. The concept of need in dental care. *Int Dent J,* 1982;32:265-70.
66. Sheiham A, Maizels J, Maizels A. New composite indicators of dental health. *Community Dent Health,* 1987; 4:407-14.
67. Marcenes W, Sheiham A. Composite indicators of dental health: functioning teeth and the number of sound-equivalent teeth (T-Health). *Community Dent Oral Epidemiol,* 1993; 21: 374-8.
68. Pinto VG. Identificação de problemas . In: Pinto VG. *Saúde Bucal Coletiva.* 4. ed. São Paulo: Ed. Santos, 2000.
69. Bönecker M, Marcenes W, Sheiham A, Guedes-Pinto AC, Walter LRF. Redução na prevalência e severidade de cárie dentária em bebês. *J Bras Odontop e Odontol Bebê,* 2000;3:334-40.
70. Mc Donald SP, Sheiham A. The distribution of caries on different tooth surfaces at varying levels of caries – a compilation of data from 18 previous studies. *Community Dental Health,* 1992;9:39-48.
71. Cohen LK. The emerging field of oral health-related quality of life outcomes research. *In*: Slade GD. *Measuring oral health and quality of life.* Chapel Hill: University of North Carolina, Dental Ecology, 1997.
72. Locker D, Miller Y. Subjectively reported oral healthstatus in an adult population. *Community Dent Oral Epidemiol,* 1994; 22:425-30.
73. Slade GD. The oral health impact profile. *In:* Slade GD. *Measuring oral health and quality of life.* Chapel Hill: University of North Carolina, Dental Ecology, 1997.
74. Walter LRF, Ferelle A, Hokama N, Pelanda, VLG, Franco MPS, Lega R. Cárie em crianças de 0 a 30 meses de idade e sua relação com hábitos alimentares. *Enc Bras Odontol,* 1987;5:129-136.
75. Bezerra ACB. Estudo clínico-epidemiológico da prevalência de cárie em crianças pré-escolares de 12 a 48 meses de idade. São Paulo, 1990. 121 p. Tese (Doutorado em Odontopediatria) - Faculdade de Odontologia da Universidade de São Paulo.
76. Morita MC, Walter LRF, Guillain M. Prévalence de la carie dentaire chez des enfants Brésiliens de 0 à 36 mois. J d' *Odonto-Stomatol Pédiatrie,* 1993;3:19-28.
77. Mattos Graner RO, Rontani RMP, Gavião MBD, Bocatto HCAR. Caries prevalence in 6-36-month old Brazilian children. *Community Dent Health,* 1996; 13: 96-98.
78. Bönecker MJS, Guedes-Pinto AC, Walter LRF. Prevalência, distribuição e grau de afecção de cárie dentária em crianças de 0 a 36 meses de idade. *Rev Assoc Paul Cir Dent,* 1997; 51: 535-539.
79. Carvalho JC, Mestrinho HD, Bezerra AC, Maltz M. Preschool child dental health status in the Federal District of Brazil. *Caries Res,* 1996;30:300.
80. Freire MCM, Melo RB, Silva SA. Dental caries prevalence in relation to socioeconomic status of nursery school children in Goiânia-GO, Brazil. *Community Dent Oral Epidemiol,* 1996;24:357-361.
81. Cerqueira L M. Estudo da dieta, da utilização de medidas preventivas e da prevalência de cárie dentária em crianças de 0 a 36 meses na cidade de Natal. Natal, 1998. 88p. Dissertação (Mestrado em

Odontologia Preventiva e Social) – Faculdade de Odontologia da Universidade Federal do Rio Grande do Norte.
82. Dini EL, Holt RD, Bedi R. Prevalence and severity of caries in 3-12-year-old children from three districts with different fluoridation histories in Araraquara, SP, Brazil. *Community Dent Health,* 1998; 15(1):44-8.
83. Fraiz F.C. Estudo dos fatores associados a cárie dentária em crianças que recebem atenção odontológica precoce. São Paulo, 1998. 108p. Tese (Doutorado em Odontopediatria) Faculdade de Odontologia da Universidade de São Paulo.
84. Detogni AM. De volta às origens. *Rev ABO Nac,* 1994;2:138-148.
85. Pinto V.G. *Estudo epidemiológico sobre prevalência de cárie dental em crianças de 3 a 14 anos:* Brasil, 1993. Brasília: Sesi-DN, 1996. 53p.
86. Tomita NE, Bijella VT, Lopes ES, Franco LF. Prevalência de cárie dentária em crianças da faixa etária de 0 a 6 anos matriculadas em creches: importância de fatores socioeconômicos. *Rev Saúde Pública,* 1996;30:413-20.
87. Arias SMB, Brandão AMM, Nogueira AJS. Prevalência de cárie em bebês de 0-3 anos. *RGO,* 1997;45:163-9.
88. Paula MPG, Dadalto ECV. Prevalência de cárie em crianças de 0 a 36 meses de idade. *Rev ABO Nac,* 2000;8:86-91.
89. Bönecker M, Marcenes W, Sheiham A. Caries reductions between 1995, 1997 and 1999 in preschool children in Diadema, Brazil. *Int J Paed Dent,* 2002;12:183-188.
90. Cleaton-Jones PE, Richardson BD, Mc Innes PM, Fatti LP. Dental caries in South African white children aged 1-5 years. *Community Dent Oral Epidem,* 1978;6:78-81.
91. Alaluusua S, Malmivirata R. Early plaque accumulation – a sign for caries risk in young children. *Community Dent Oral Epidemiol,* 1994;22:273-6.
92. Hugoson A, Koch G, Bergendal T, Hallonsten A-L, Laurell L, Lundgren D, Nyman J-E. Oral health of individuals aged 3-80 years in Jönköping, Sweden, in 1973 and 1983. *Swed Dent J,* 1985;10 (3):175-94.
93. Holt R.D. Caries in the preschool child: British trends. *J Dent,* 1990;18:296-299.
94. Wendt L-K, Hallonsten A-L, Koch G. Oral health in preschool children living in Sweden. Part II. *Swed Dent J,* 1992;16(1/2):41-9.
95. Silver DH. A comparison of 3-years-olds' caries experience in 1973, 1981 and 1989 in a Hertfordshire town, related to family behavior and social class. *Br Dent J,* 1992;172:191-197.
96. Grindefjord M, Dahllöf G, Nilsson B, Modéer T. Stepwise prediction of dental caries in children up to 3,5 years of age. *Caries Res,* 1996;30:256-266.
97. Kaste LM, Selwitz RH, Oldakowski RJ, Brunelle JA, Winn DM, Brown LJ. Coronal caries in the primary and permanent dentition of children and adolescents 1-17 years of age: United States, 1988-1991. *J Dent Res,* 1996;75: 631-641. Número especial.
98. Seow WK, Amaratunge A, Sim R, Wan A. Prevalence of caries in urban Australian aborigines aged 1-3,5 years. *Pediatr Dent,* 1999;21:91-96.
99. Levantamento epidemiológico em saúde bucal – cárie dental – capitais, índice CPO por região e UF e idade. Período: 1996. SUS. Ministério da Saúde, Brasil.
100. Pinto VG. Projeto de levantamento epidemiológico nacional em saúde bucal não tem consistência. *Jornal da APCD,* 1996; p.15.
101. Dini EL, Holt RD, Bedi R. Prevalence and severity of caries in 3-12 year-old children from three districts with different fluoridation histories in Araraquara, SP, Brazil. Community Dental Health, 1998; 15:44-48.
102. Ministério da Saúde. Resultados da fluoretação da água de consumo pela fundação SESP, 1993. Quadros. Pinto VG. Epidemiologia das Doenças Bucais no Brasil p.29-41. In: *ABOPREV Promoção de Saúde Bucal: São Paulo.* Artes Médicas, 1997.
103. Viegas Y, Viegas AR. Prevalência de cárie dental em Barretos, SP, Brasil, após dezesseis anos de fluoretação da água de abastecimento público. *Rev Saúde Pública,* 1988;22:25-35.
104. Prefeitura Municipal de Blumenau. Relatório das Atividades; 1968.
105. Levantamento epidemiológico de cárie dental em escolares de Blumenau, 1998. Relatório final; 1998.
106. Viegas Y, Viegas AR. Prevalência de cárie dental na cidade de Campinas, SP, Brasil, depois de quatorze anos de fluoretação da água de abastecimento público. *Rev Assoc Paul Cir Dent,* 1985; 39:272-76.
107. Boletim epidemiológico de saúde oral de Curitiba. 1997, Ano 1, n.1, 2º semestre.

108. Levantamento epidemiológico das condições de saúde bucal do Estado de São Paulo – Município de Diadema sob supervisão da FSP-USP Dir II, 1997.
109. Marcenes W, Freyslebeng R, Peres MA. The contribution of changing diagnostic criteria toward the reduction of caries between 1971 and 1997 in children attending the same school in Florianópolis, Brazil. *Community Dent Oral Epidemiol,* 2001;449-455.
110. Ogawa AT. Índice CPO-D em crianças de 7 a 12 anos em 1981, 1987 e 1992 em Londrina – Paraná. *In:* Pinto VG. Epidemiologia das Doenças Bucais no Brasil p.29-41. *In: ABOPREV Promoçao de Saúde Bucal.* Artes Médicas, 1997.
111. Moreira BW, Pereira AC, Oliveira SP. Avaliação da prevalência de cárie dentária em escolares de localidade urbana da Região Sudeste do Brasil. *Rev Saúde Pública,* 1996;30:280-84.
112. Kalamatianos PA, Naressi WG. Estudo comparativo do índice CPO antes e depois do advento da educação sanitária nas escolas da rede municipal da cidade de São José dos Campos/SP. *RGO,* 1988; 36:327-30.
113. Arcieri RM, Carvalho ML, Gonçalves LMG, Almeida HA, Pereira ALC, Oliveira EM. Estudo comparativo da prevalência de cárie dentária após 10 (dez) anos de adição de flúor nas águas de abastecimento público de Uberlândia – MG. *Rev Paul Odontol,* 1986;82:46-55.
114. Bönecker M, Cleaton-Jones PE. Trends in dental caries in Latin American and Caribbean 5 and 11-13-year-old children: a systematic review. *Community Dent Oral Epidemiol,* 2003;31:152-7.
115. WHO Web Page – www.whocollab.ed.mah.se
116. Brathall D, Hansen Peterson G, Sundberg H. Reasons for the caries decline: what do experts believe? *Eur J Oral Sci,* 1996; 104:416-22.
117. Downer MC. The caries decline. A comment in light of the UK experience. *Eur J Oral Sci,* 1996;104:433-35.
118. Sheiham A. Impact of dental treatment on the incidence of dental caries in children and adults. *Community Dent Oral Epidemiol,* 1997;25:104-12
119. Freyslebeng R, Peres MA, Marcenes W. Dental caries prevalence and mean DMFT among schoolchildren between 1971 to 1997, Brazil. *Rev Saúde Pública,* 2000; 34:304-8.
120. Downer MC. Caries experience and sucrose availability: an analysis of the relationship in the United Kingdom over fifty years. *Community Dent Health,* 1999; 16:18-21.
121. Birkeland JM, Hangejorden O, Ramm von der Fehr, F. Some factors associated with the caries decline among Norwegian children and adolescents: age specific and cohort analysis. *Caries Res,* 2000;34:109-16.
122. Cleaton-Jones PE, Chosa CKA, Hargraves JA, Fatti LP. Dental caries and social factors in 12 years old South African children. *Community Dent Oral Epidemiol,* 1994; 22:25-29.
123. Treasure ET, Dever VG. Relationship of caries with socioeconomic status in 14 year old children from communities with different fluoride stories. *Community Dent Oral Epidemiol,* 1994; 22:226-30.
124. Schou L, Uitenbroe KD. Social and behavioral indicators of caries experience in 5 year old children. *Community Dent Oral Epidemiol,* 1995; 23: 276-81.
125. Jones L. Behavioral and environmental influences on health. In: Katz J, Peberdy A. *Promoting Health. Knowledge and Pratice.* London: The Open University; 1977.
126. MacKeown T. *The role of medicine: dream, mirage or nemesis.* Cambridge: Nuffield. Provincial Hospitals Trust.
127. Moysés ST, Watt R. Promoção de saúde bucal. Definições. *In:* Buischi YP. *Promoção de Saúde Bucal no Consultório Odontológico. São Paulo: Artes Médicas, 2000.*

Chapter **2**

Public Health Approaches to Promoting Periodontal Health

Aubrey Sheiham

Introduction

Approaches to preventing and controlling periodontal disease have changed markedly. Systematic reviews of the effectiveness and efficiency of individualised dental health education approaches to change oral hygiene have been relatively ineffective in making sustained changes in toothbrushing. The reason for the unacceptably high failure rates in changing behaviours is the failure to recognise the social contextual factors that are related to health behaviours in general.

There are other reasons for the lack of success in promoting periodontal health.

- The models of the life history of periodontal disease that have been outlined since the 1970s by Socransky, Goodson and Hafferjee suggest that most periodontal inflammation does not progress to severe destructive periodontal disease. Therefore concepts of risk and susceptibility need revising.
- The changes in concepts of what is potentially important periodontal pathology have lead to a re-evaluation of the importance of periodontal disease as a dental public health problem.
- The lay views of about the relative unimportance of periodontal disease have been substantiated. Gingival inflammation seldom causes discomfort, social embarrassment or loss of function. Instead of expecting people to know that they have periodontal disease, dentists need to review their ideas and place more emphasis on the social aspects of periodontal inflammation such as oral malodour, gingival recession and bleeding and redness.

This chapter will review the concepts and the causes of periodontal diseases that are relevant for public health and the public health approaches to their control.

Models of periodontal diseases

The natural history of periodontal disease progression is not as simple as suggested previously. The old 'Continuous Progression' model of periodontal disease considers that gingivitis progress to periodontitis; then the slow loss of attachment and its bony support progresses continuously until the tooth is non-functional. Such a model suggests that once a person has periodontal disease only continuous treatment will prevent the inevitable progress of the destructive lesion to severe periodontitis. There is little evidence to support this model. The continuous progression model has been challenged by the 'burst' model.

Not all gingivitis progresses to periodontitis. The 'burst' theory incorporated the concept of 'contained gingivitis' and 'stable gingivitis' classify gingival inflammation which is limited to the gingivae. Many inflamed gingival sites remain free of destructive periodontal disease for a lifetime. Other sites experience one or more bursts of destructive disease followed by a period of repair or remission. Few sites develop advanced destructive disease.

Epidemiological surveys in diverse populations show that contrary to earlier reports, susceptibility to advanced periodontal disease is not universal; the prevalence of destructive periodontal diseases is considerably lower than previously estimated and the public's periodontal health is improving In particular the worldwide prevalence of severe periodontal disease is very low and rates of progression of periodontal destruction, very slow.

The two main changes in knowledge about periodontal disease, are:

- A small proportion of persons exhibit severe widespread periodontitis. Mild gingivitis is common and most adults demonstrate some loss of bony support and loss of probing attachment.
- There is consensus that severe periodontal disease occurs in a few teeth in a relatively small proportion of people in any given age cohort, the proportion affected increases with age.
- Periodontitis is not the major cause of tooth loss in adults.

So contrary to the view that destructive periodontal was widespread and that everyone is susceptible to advanced destructive periodontal disease, current epidemiological evidence indicates that the severity and rate of the loss of periodontal support in the majority of populations does not lead to significant psychological and social impacts related to gingival recession and mobility and much tooth loss.

Factors that may cause the conversion of gingivitis to periodontitis

According to the burst models the indications for treatment of affected sites are no longer clear unless the reduction of plaque could shorten or decrease the intensity of the burst. Indeed, the dogma that all gingivitis must be eliminated and any periodontal pocket must be treated should be seriously questioned. Inflammatory changes of the gingivae could be considered an indicator of a healthy defence mechanism. Treating people with periodontal pockets but who are not in an active phase of the disease is analogous to treating a patient for pneumonia who has a radiolucency now but how had the disease some years earlier. The presence of a periodontal pocket does not necessarily indicate active disease. A pocket may be a legacy of past disease and is not more likely to breakdown further than a site without a pocket. So periodontal treatment may not be necessary and could be harmful. Conventional measures such as root planing and periodontal surgery have been shown to lead to deepening of periodontal pockets of 4 mm or less.

Assessment of those at risk

An important part of planning dental care systems is diagnosing those with active disease and detecting cases that are likely to develop disease in future. There are no reliable markers of periodontal disease activity nor predictors of who will develop periodontitis. Neither is it known which sites will progress from gingival inflammation to periodontitis. Some of the clinical signs used to indicate disease have been questioned. Indeed one may question whether gingival inflammation, commonly called gingivitis, is a disease. Periodontal health is considered to be the absence of gingivitis, no loss of attachment and anatomically perfect gingival contours; the absence of disease and its consequences.

The new concepts of periodontal diseases suggest that many gingival sites remain free of destructive periodontal disease for a lifetime. Some sites experience one or more bursts of destructive disease followed by a period of repair or remission. The remission following a burst may be permanent or intermittent. These new concepts of periodontal diseases require a radical change in ideas on diagnosis, screening and methods of treatment.

The difficulties in defining periodontal health, the erratic nature of destructive disease, and the poor sensitivity and specificity of methods of predicting destructive disease suggests that screening for periodontal disease is not justified.

There is a very small minority of people who develop rapidly progressing periodontal disease. At present there is insufficient evidence to identify them. The prime objective of screening is to detect disease at an earlier stage than would occur with people presenting with the illness, on the assumption that earlier treatment would alter the natural history of the disease in a significant proportion. Despite encouraging developments in the bacteriology and immunological aspects relating to periodontal diseases there remain major gaps in knowledge before screening can be recommended. Neither is there sufficient evidence on prognostic indicators of severe periodontal disease activity nor of future destructive periodontal disease. Research is progressing to develop indicators. At present no biotechnology on prognostic indicators is available for use in the practice setting. Therefore, population screening for periodontal destruction in future life is not yet feasible.

Plaque and periodontal disease

A relationship, which has stood the test of time, is that between plaque and periodontal disease. In addition, smoking is known to affect periodontal disease. The aetiology of chronic inflammatory periodontal diseases can be considered in terms of the microorganisms involved, the local oral environmental factors other than bacteria, and the role played by the host defence systems.

There are three main theories on the role of plaque bacteria in periodontal disease. The "specific", the "non-specific plaque hypothesis" and the "ecological plaque hypothesis".

- The specific plaque hypothesis states that a very limited number of organisms are actively involved in causing disease.
- The non-specific plaque hypothesis says that many of the heterogeneous mixture of organisms in plaque play a role in disease.
- Marsh challenged the dichotomy between the theories since plaque-mediated diseases, while not necessarily having a totally specific etiology, do show evidence of specificity. Marsh proposed a unifying "ecological plaque hypothesis". This hypothesis proposes that a change in a key environmental factor triggers a shift in the balance of the resident plaque microflora.

The direct cause of gingivitis and periodontitis is the accumulation of microbial plaque on the cervical region of the teeth and its extension apically along the root surface. Both gingivitis and periodontitis appears to be caused by a progression of sequentially changing species, but the flora in the two conditions is not the same.

The new concepts of the progression of periodontal disease appear to challenge the relationship between the quantity of

periodontal pocket deeper than 3mm must be treated should be seriously questioned. Treating people with periodontal pockets but who are not in an active phase of the disease is analogous to treating a patient for pneumonia who has a radiolucency now but had the disease some years earlier. In addition to such criticisms of treatment some commonly recommended treatments such as root planing have been shown to be unnecessary. Such treatment could indeed be harmful. Conventional measures such as root planing and periodontal surgery lead to deepening of periodontal pockets of 4mm or less and loss of attachment.

Surgery and root planing are of questionable benefit and they deserve little place in any public dental health programme.

The long-term value of removing calculus is not supported by evidence from clinical trials, and there is some doubt about the usefulness of removing calculus, particularly in groups with low calculus scores. Professional cleaning at 6 or 3-monthly intervals does not significantly improve periodontal health. Other dogmas have also been evaluated and found wanting. They include:

- if teeth are not kept plaque-free after treatment periodontal disease will inevitably return with progressive loss of attachment.
- the deeper the pockets the poorer the prognosis.
- advanced periodontal cannot be stopped by treatment.
- non-surgical treatment is ineffective for treating deep pockets.

In a state-of-the-science review of mechanical oral hygiene practices, Frandsen (1986) came to some important conclusions which have implications for public health aspects of periodontal disease. The conclusions are:

- There is no scientific evidence that one specific toothbrush type and design is more superior at removing plaque.
- The roll technique of toothbrushing is the least effective of removing plaque; no single method was superior to other methods.
- Daily use of floss by children with healthy gingiva can be damaging.
- There is no scientific justification for recommending forced irrigation devices.
- Well-motivated and instructed people can clean their mouths adequately with most of the available oral hygiene aids and techniques.
- The efficiency of personal, mechanical oral hygiene practices is more likely to be enhanced through an understanding of factors determining performance rather than by attempts to improve aids and techniques.
- The optimal frequency and starting age for scaling and polishing has not been determined. The 6-month interval is unsubstantiated and is too general a recommendation.
- Regular instrumentation and polishing should not be carried out at disease-free sites.
- The role of root planing in preventing re-infection of the subgingival area is questionable.
- Scaling, polishing, root planing, and surgical treatment of shallow periodontal pockets results in permanent loss of attachment.

Public health strategies

The changes in concepts and treatment mentioned have considerable implications for the future practice of dentistry in general and for public health approaches to periodontal diseases in particular. The most important implication is the reassessment of periodontal diseases as a public health problem in general and a dental public health problem in particular. For a disease to be considered a public health problem requiring action it should fulfil certain conditions. These are:

- disease must be widespread (if it is uncommon it must be serious);
- consequences (impact) to the community and to individuals are severe;
- effective methods must be available to prevent, alleviate, or cure the disease;
- costs to the community and to individuals is great.

Although severe periodontal disease is not widespread, the fact that the costs of treating the disease are high because of the organization of dental care, qualifies it as a dental public problem. In addition the symptoms of periodontal diseases such as bleeding, halitosis, gingival recession and tooth loss have an impact on many people. And we have sufficient information to control the common forms of the disease.

Goals for periodontal disease control

The goal of a plaque free mouth is both unrealistic and unnecessary.

A reasonable goal for periodontal disease control is to achieve a level of plaque which is compatible with a rate of periodontal destruction which will retain teeth essential for an socially and personally acceptable dentition for a lifetime; one that does not cause handicaps.

Reduction in the quantity of dental plaque will reduce the severity of gingival inflammation and the probability of destructive periodontal diseases. Calculus does not have a major role in the pathogenesis of periodontal diseases. The clinical basis, as distinct from social reasons, for calculus removal is unjustified.

Strategies for controlling periodontal diseases

The plan for controlling periodontal disease has three components:

- A population strategy for altering life practices and in particular oral cleaning effectiveness to reduce the dental plaque level of the community.
- A secondary prevention strategy to detect and treat people with destructive periodontal disease.
- A high-risk strategy for bringing preventive and therapeutic care to individuals at special risk.

Population strategy

A reduction in plaque in the general population can be achieved by using the information on factors affecting tooth cleaning behaviour. Because tooth cleaning is associated with grooming and personal hygiene and religious beliefs, most people do clean their teeth regularly. The objective of health education is to improve the effectiveness of tooth cleaning behaviour. Since tooth cleaning is part of general hygiene behaviour, programs directed at improving tooth cleanliness should be incorporated in health education directed at improving body cleanliness and grooming. These programs should emphasize lay competence, be supportive and non-mystifying, and should not 'blame the victim'.

The health education programme should incorporate methods and concepts which will encourage the maintenance of an adequate level of oral cleanliness without professional reinforcement. The programme should therefore stress the following factors;

- Tooth cleaning behaviour is part of general cleanliness.
- Relevance of behaviours.
- Social acceptability of tooth cleaning methods.

- Easily incorporated into daily activities.
- The simplicity of tooth cleaning.
- Feedback methods to assess whether cleaning is being done effectively.

The programs should contain the following components:

- A community-wide approach incorporating the principles of integration with general health education, diversity of educational approaches and community participation in planning and implementation.
- Community leader education to improve health behaviour through the better understanding and involvement of leaders of public opinion. They act as role models and their management and organisational skills help to implement preventive strategies.
- Public education to increase awareness and knowledge of good hygiene behaviour by educating all age groups in a continuing and consistent programme.
- Mass-media methods to increase community awareness of body hygiene and tooth cleanliness, the availability of oral hygiene aids and plaque disclosing agents to be used for feedback.
- Environmental changes – the encouragement of health-promoting behaviour may be achieved by modifying the environment, e.g. improvements in hygiene at schools and in the workplace, provision of washing facilities and the introduction of marketing practices which encourage the sale of good oral hygiene aids at low cost.
- Professional education to improve tooth-cleaning instruction by professional personnel. Teachers, nursery school attendants, health visitors, nurses, doctors, dentists and other dental personnel and health educators should be provided with specific oral hygiene education so that they will provide accurate information and set good examples.
- Smoking cessation integration with general health education and health promotion.

The objective of all informal and formal dental health education is to foster negotiation and collaboration so that patients might be helped to make informed choices. It involves acquisition of knowledge and understanding and the development of skills for self-care. The aim is to elicit, to facilitate and to support the maintenance of effective oral cleaning practices. To achieve the aims and objective, a planned consistent, integrated series of strategies should be adopted.

The plan should be based on the following concepts:

- Integration and use of common risk factor approach. Dental health education should be integrated with general health education into the activities of teachers, all health workers, community leaders, trade unionists, sportspeople and all members of the dental team. Oral cleanliness education should be integrated with general health education about body cleanliness, grooming and self-esteem. Smoking cessation is pivotal to improving oral hygiene.
- Diverse educational approaches. An oral cleanliness education program must incorporate a number of diverse educational approaches because individuals have different needs and are at differing stages of behaviour change. Each group in the community responds differently to any given approach. Changing behaviour necessitates the application of several methods differently to various groups. Individual instruction, group discussion, mass media and community development methods can be used. These educational methods must be cumulative

and consistent. There is no best method. A given combination of methods may be effective for some people but not for others. Encourage modelling and reinforcement.
- Early intervention. The earlier the intervention in the health career, the more effective is the result. Various influences and agencies impinge on the health careers of people. The influence of primary and secondary socialization is paramount in establishing toothbrushing habits. Stress imitation of mothers and teachers. Toothbrushing is both health related and health directed. Habit, grooming, cleanliness and prevention are reasons for brushing.

Participation

Community, public and staff participation in the planning process should increase the probability of success. To foster negotiation between the learner and the practitioner involves the participation of the patient in the education process. Ask people about the practicalities of incorporating the recommendations into their daily routines.

- Encourage self-efficacy.
- Make healthier choices the easier choices.

Evaluation is needed to assess whether the programme is achieving the aims, whether it is doing so effectively and efficiently and whether their planning methods are sound.

Secondary prevention strategy

Assessment of periodontal treatment needs and periodontal status

Information on the treatment needs of populations are required to quantify the resources required to prevent and treat periodontal diseases. Such data also provide a rational basis for setting goals and to monitor the effectiveness of current strategies.

Treatment

Oral hygiene education is the most important aspect of periodontal treatment for those with signs of periodontal disease. In most people, toothbrushing alone will be adequate to control dental plaque and reverse early periodontal disease. In some people at certain sites in the mouth, dental floss with or without other mechanical aids will be necessary.

Health education programs including oral cleanliness should stress the following toothbrushing guidelines:

- Emphasise effectiveness rather than frequency – brushing more than twice daily does not improve periodontal health unless it is done effectively.
- The scrub method should be encouraged.
- Hold the brush with a finger (pen grip), not a fist grip.
- The brush ends should be directed at the gum margins.
- Make sure all the teeth surfaces are cleaned.
- Use a short-headed nylon toothbrush.

Removal of gross calculus and factors favouring plaque retention will facilitate oral cleanliness. Surgical treatment and root planing are not justified.

When the person has learnt adequate oral hygiene skills, recall intervals for re-assessment can be steadily increased from to twelve and eighteen months.

High risk strategy

There are a small number of people who will have severe progressive destructive periodontal disease despite effective tooth-cleaning practices. In these cases appropriate antimicrobial therapy could be used to change the bacterial flora in the pockets.

People with AIDS present special periodontal problems. The manifestation of periodontal lesions is often severe.

The other groups of people who would require a high-risk strategy are those with medical or sociopsychological conditions which would be affected by periodontal disease. Both the periodontal and the medical high-risk groups should be assessed by socio-psychological as well as clinical and bacteriological methods because there is growing evidence that psychological states can affect the immune response and alter the bacterial flora of the mouth. The established subgingival flora can be affected in the short term but is remarkably robust in the long term.

It is apparent that a combination of a population strategy, a secondary prevention strategy and a high-risk strategy is essential to achieve the objective of maintaining a functional, aesthetically and socially acceptable natural dentition for the lifespan of most people. The balance of effort should be heavily weighted towards the population strategy. If that strategy is adopted the need for treatment will be reduced and treatment will be more successful.

The adoption of a population strategy will be socially and economically more acceptable for a number of reasons. Firstly, periodontal disease is not considered an important public health problem. Epidemiological evidence supports that consideration. These conclusions are relevant to underdeveloped countries because, although gingivitis and shallow pocketing are common, few people lose teeth because of periodontal diseases. There is no doubt that inflammatory changes of the periodontium are widespread in most populations but the need to treat every inflamed periodontal site must be seriously questioned. Secondly, the dentist-based approach is very expensive. Thirdly, the population strategy approach can be incorporated into health education programs concerned with controlling chronic disease related to smoking, such as cardiovascular and lung diseases and school-based education programs on personal hygiene. Therefore the cost will be low and the effectiveness should be high. Fourthly, the strategy will be continuous and will not rely on campaigns and fear-arousing victim-blaming methods.

The most important implication from the analysis of relevant strategies for controlling periodontal diseases is that, since the diseases are dirt and hygiene related diseases which will be altered by improvements in general body cleanliness, efforts should be integrated with general hygiene programs carried out by primary health workers and teachers.

Manpower implications

As the most important aspect of a public health approach to preventing and controlling periodontal diseases is health promotion strategies to improve general body cleanliness and oral cleanliness, an integrated approach with general hygiene programs carried out by primary health workers and teachers, the dental personnel should have education and organizational skills. A well trained dental health educator could fulfill that role. They should teach teachers, nursery school attendants, health visitors, nurses, doctors, dentists and other dental personnel and health educators.

Dental health educators are the most valuable ancillary in periodontal health programs. They should integrate their activities with those of the health education/promotion department.

The treatment and care of the vast majority of people with periodontal diseases can be done by dental ancillaries. Dentists are not required for treating routine cases. Their role is to diagnose and treatment plan.

Evaluation and monitoring of prevention, treatment and trends in periodontal health should be carried out routinely by an epidemiologist.

References

1. Abegg A, Marcenes W, Croucherm R, Sheiham A. The relationship between tooth cleaning behaviour and flexibility of working time schedule *J Clin Periodontol,* 1999; 26:448-452.
2. Abegg C, Croucher R, Marcenes WS, Sheiham A. How do routines of daily activities and flexibility of daily activities affect tooth-cleaning behavior? *J Public Health Dentistry,* 2000; 60 (3); 154-158.
3. Antczak-Boukoms A. Natural history of periodontitis and a review of technologies to prevent and treat it. *J Dent Educ,* 1994; 58:625-640.
4. Burt BA. Public health implications of recent research in periodontal diseases. *J Public Health Dentistry,* 1988; 48:252-256.
5. Frandsen, A. *Public Health Aspects of Periodontal Disease.* Chicago: Quintesence Publ. Co. 1984.
6. Frandsen, A. Mechanical oral hygiene practises. *In: Dental plaque control measures and oral hygiene practices,* 1986. eds. Loe, H. Kleinman D.V. p. 93-116. Oxford: IRL Press.
7. Jenkins WMM. Papapanou PN. *Epidemiology of periodontal disease in children and adolescents.* Periodontol, 2000 26:16-32.
8. Kay, E. Locker, D. *Effectiveness of oral health promotion: a review.* Health Education Authority.
9. Lang N, Joss A, Orsanic T, Gusberti FA, Siegrist BE. Bleeding on probing. A predictor for the progression of periodontal disease? *J Clin Periodont* 1986, 13:590-596.
10. Listgarten, MA. Why do epidemiological data have no diagnostic value? In: *Periodontology Today,* ed B. Guggheim, 1988, pp. 59-67 Basel: S. Karger AG.
11. Loesche WJ. Chemotherapy of dental plaque infections. *Oral Sci Res* 1976; 9:65-107.
12. Marsh PD. Microbial ecology of dental plaqque and its significance in health and disease. *Adv Dent Res* 1994; 8 (2):263-271.
13. Moysés ST, Moysés SJ, Watt RG. Sheiham A. (2002) The impact of health promotion schools policies on oral health of 12 year olds. *Health Promotion Internationale* (In Press).
14. Page, RC. Current understanding of the etiology and progression of periodontal disease. *International Dental Journal,* 36,153-161, 1996.
15. Papapanou PN. Periodontal Diseasses: Epidemiology, 1996. Ann Periodontol 1:1 30.
16. Pilot, T. Analysis of the overall effectiveness of treatment of periodontal disease. *In: Efficacy of treatment procedures in periodontics,* ed D. Shanley, 1981, p. 213-230 Chicago: Quintessence Publ. Co.
17. Pilot, T. Implementation of preventive periodontal programs at a community level. *In: Public Health Aspects of Periodontal Disease,* ed A. Frandsen, 1984; p. 181-196 Chicago: Quintessence Publ. Co.
18. Pilot T. Implications for health screening and public health planning. *In:* Johnson NW. ed. Risk markers for oral diseases. *Periodontal diseases. Markers of disease susceptibility and activity.* Cambridge University Press, 1991.
19. Rose, G. *The Strategy of Preventive Medicine.* Oxford: Oxford University Press, 1992.
20. Shanley, D. *Efficacy of treatment procedures in periodontics.* Chicago: Quintessence, 1981.
21. Sheiham, A. Screening for periodontal disease, *J Clin Periodont,* 1978;5, 237-245.
22. Sheiham, A. Public health aspects of periodontal diseases in Europe. *J Clin Periodontol,* 1991;18, 362-369.
23. Sheiham, A. Is the chemical prevention of gingivitis necessary to prevent severe periodontitis? *Periodontology* 2000, 1997;15, 15-24.
24. Sheiham, A. & Watt RG. The common risk factor approach: a rational approach for promoting oral health. *Community Dent Oral Epidemiol,* 2000; 28,399-406.
25. Socransky SS, Haffajee AD, Goodson JM, Lindhe J. New concepts of destructive periodontal disease. *J Clin Periodontol,* 11, 1984;21-32.
26. Wennströmm JL. What is a clinical healthy

periodontium? In: Guggeheim B. ed. Periodontology Today, Basel: Krager, 1988, p.1-5.
27. Wennström JL, Papapanou PN, Gröndahl K. A model for decision making regarding periodontal treeatment needs. *J Clin Periodontol,* 1990; 17:217-222.

Chapter 3

Traumatic Dental Injury

Wagner Marcenes

Introduction

Promoting oral health throughout reduction of traumatic dental injuries (TDI) is a challenging experience. Contrary to other common oral conditions such as dental caries, which is related to diet, in particular to sugar consumption, TDI is related to a number of harmful non-violent or violent incidents. Thus, a problem-oriented approach must be adopted. This means there is not one receipt to apply to all circumstances. Each activity related to TDI asks for a problem-oriented approach. Therefore, a successful health promotion strategy to reduce the prevalence of traumatic dental injuries should be based on epidemiological data on the location, injury events and intention at local level, as they will vary in accordance to local habits. For example, there is no point in focus efforts on home and school physical environment, if the injury events are occurring in the street. Similarly, it would be ineffective to focus on providing mouthguards to children, if only a small proportion of dental injuries are related to playing sports.

Location should include (1) home, (2) school, (3) work, (4) street/road/pavement and (5) leisure areas. Ten major injury events could be derived from the literature. They were (1) physical leisure activities, (2) playing with others, (3) inappropriate using of teeth (i.e.: use of teeth as a tool to fix devices), (4) eating, (5) traffic accident, (6) violent incident, (7) illness, (8) health care accident (Adverse effect of medical care), (9) falls and (10) collisions. Major categories such as physical leisure activities included sub categories such as sports, cycling, rollerskating and diving. Sub categories such as playing football will be a more common injury event in Brasil, while iceskating will be a more frequent injury event in Scandinavian countries. Finally, intention should be assessed. This represents the role of human intent in the occurrence of the TDI event. Three intention categories were identified. They were unintentional, intentional and iatrogenic dental injury events.

Traumatic dental injury: a neglected dental public health problem

Possibly the most important health promotion strategy related to traumatic dental injury is to acknowledge that this neglected condition is a developing dental public health (Marcenes et al, 1999). A number of factors need to be taken into account when assessing whether or not a condition is a

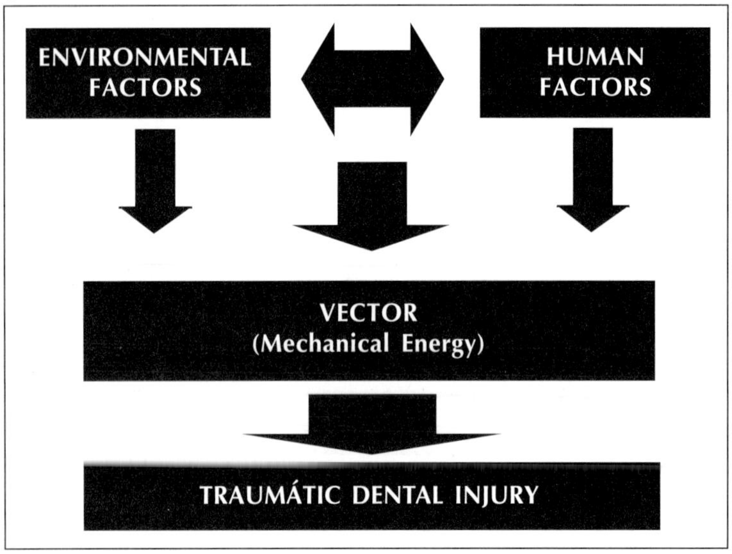

Fig. 3.1 Aetiology of traumatic dental injuries.

dental public health problem. The condition should be widespread in a population; it may be life-threatening or have a significant impact on individuals and society; and a body of knowledge should exist about its causation factors and treatment.

The prevalence of dental injuries is high (Andreasen and Andreasen, 1994). One of the few prospective research design studies, which has been carried out in Denmark, has shown that half of all children may experience at least one dental injury before leaving school (Andreasen and Ravn, 1972). Recently, a retrospective research design carefully carried out using reliable dental records from Sweden showed that 35% of 16-year-old children studied had on one or more occasions sustained dental injury (Borssen and Holm, 1997). High prevalence of dental injuries was also reported when a cross-sectional design was used; and this was probably a gross underestimation of its prevalence (Andreasen and Andreasen, 1994). Furthermore, there is some evidence that the prevalence of traumatic dental injuries is much higher in socially deprived areas than the overall prevalence in the UK. For example, the prevalence of traumatic dental injuries at the age of 14 years in two deprived areas of the UK was much higher than the overall prevalence, 43.8% in Newham (Marcenes and Murray, 2002) and 34.4% in Bury and Salford (Ref), compared to a prevalence of 17% in the UK.

Data from England also showed that contrary to the dramatic reduction in the prevalence and severity of dental caries observed in the last decades, the prevalence of TDI appears to be steady around 20%. If these trends continue, dental caries will become less prevalent than traumatic dental injuries (graph here??????). Data from Wales and Scotland show a similar pattern as the one observed in England. In Northern Ireland, the prevalence of traumatic dental injuries appears to be increasing, while the prevalence of dental caries is decreasing. Data from Newham, a deprived district in England, also demonstrate a sharp increase in the prevalence of traumatic dental injuries, 23.7% in 1995-96 and 43.8% in 1998-99.

In addition to the relatively high prevalence, dental injuries have a large impact on children's quality of life. The majority of dental injuries involve the anterior teeth (Andreasen and Andreasen, 1994), which may impose a physical and socio-psychological trauma on children. The physical trauma is well known and it does not need further discussion here. The socio-psychological trauma is less known as only one study has been carried out to assess the impact of traumatic dental injuries on daily life, using a socio-dental indicator. This study was carried out in Brasil in 204 12 to 14 year old children and confirmed that untreated fractures at the dentin level have a significant impact on the daily life of children. They affect the ability of enjoying food, tooth cleaning, smiling and showing teeth without embarrassment, maintaining an emotional state without being irritable, and socialising.

Thus, it is not surprising that children with untreated fractures at the dentin level are 20 times more likely to report impacts on their daily life than children who do not have a fracture.

It is not surprising that children with untreated fractured teeth tend to be much more unhappy with the appearance of their teeth than children without fractured teeth, 17% compared to 2.9%. In addition, children with untreated fractured teeth tend to be teased about their teeth more often than children without fractured teeth, 26.5% compared to 6.6%. This may lead to bullying, social exclusion and low self-esteem. Further studies are needed to assess the long-term socio-psychological effects of dental injuries. These studies should include measures of self esteem, inter-personal relationships, as well as education, work and marital attainment. There is a potential chain of risk from having a dental injury to the development of adverse psychological outcomes, and later in life to experience cognitive, labour and marital adversity.

In summary, traumatic dental injury is a new challenge for dental health professionals and dental health professional must acknowledge that this neglected condition needs further attention.

Traumatic dental injury is preventable

Possibly the second most important health promotion strategy related to traumatic dental injury is to acknowledge that traumatic dental injuries are preventable. Unfortunately, the traditional view of injuries as "accidents" or "random events" has resulted in the historical neglect of this health condition.

A body of knowledge exists on the aetiology of dental injury. It is well known that boys have significantly more dental injuries than girls, and that increased incisal overjet of the teeth and inadequate lip coverage are significant predisposing factors to traumatic dental injury (Andreasen and Andreasen, 1994). More distal causes of traumatic dental injuries are behavioural and environmental. Risk-taking children tend to have more dental injuries than their less risk-taking counterparts (Ref). Also, children with peer relationship problems have significantly more dental injuries than other children (Ref). In addition, hyperactive children have significantly more dental injuries than non-hyperactive children (Ref). Interestedly, children who show pro-social behaviour tend to have less dental injuries than those who show anti-social behaviour (Ref). An obvious example of environmental causes of dental injuries is an unsafe environment. High levels of deprivation have been related to dental injuries, in particular overcrowding houses (ref).

Thus, traumatic dental injuries do not occur at random, they have a cause and they are preventable. The most effective approach, based on the science of injury prevention, would target the environment rather than the behaviour. For example, a child who is more risk-taking might be more likely to fall when playing on playground equipment. However if the surface underneath the equipment is designed to absorb the energy of the fall, the injury can be prevented without changing the behaviour. Despite near universal knowledge that high sugar consumption results in dental caries, a high number of children remain consuming high amount of sugar in most developed countries in the world. Explanatory models that link risk-taking and prevention to rational processes such as knowledge, social norms, behavioural intentions, cannot fully explain the continued oral health risk behaviour of high sugar alcohol and tobacco consumption observed worldwide. In addition, a large number of doctors, dentists, nurses and other health professionals smoke. Furthermore, evidence from systematic reviews has confirmed that health education fail to change behaviour (ref). Thus, unless innovative and evidence based conceptions of risk and risk prevention are developed, environmental changes seems to be a more effective strategy than trying to alter children's behaviour, especially when sustained behaviour changes in the high-risk groups is what would be needed to effectively decrease dental injury through this approach.

A health promotion strategy to traumatic dental injuries involves three levels:

- The prevention of potential harmful events.
- The prevention of dental injuries when a harmful event cannot or should not be prevented.
- The prevention of the biological and socio-psychological impacts of dental injuries by optimal care.

Dental health professionals may significantly contribute to health promotion strategies related to traumatic dental injuries at all three levels. However, to focus efforts on the first and second level may reduce the prevalence of traumatic dental injuries and avoid the high financial cost of their treatment. Undesirable events such as a violent incident should be prevented. However, physical leisure activities are part of the health promotion message for good general health and should not be avoided to prevent traumatic dental injuries. In this case, the focus should be on the prevention of dental injuries when the event happened.

Main traumatic dental injury events

Worldwide, physical leisure activities, violence and traffic "accidents" tend to account for most traumatic dental injuries among adolescents. Playing with others, eating and inappropriate use of teeth also contribute to have a traumatic dental injury, but to a less extent. "Falls" and "collisions" tend to be the most prevalent injury events reported in the literature. This cover up the actual injury events, which may be a violent incident and it does not help to design a health promotion strategy. For example, falls from pushing is a minor form of violence that should not be recorded as "falls" as in most studies. Also, it is common for a child to be pushed against another child or object, in particular the school water tap. If intention is assessed these events would be recorded as bullying, a minor violence, rather than collision. Of concern is the high proportion of children who tend to reported "unknown cause". Often a child tends to report "unknown cause" when the damage is due to violence. Thus, it is possible that the role of violence in the occurrence of traumatic dental injuries has been terribly underestimated. (ref).

Traffic related health promotion strategies

Traffic related health promotion strategies provide examples of successful strategies in developed countries. A combination of engineering, enforcement through legislation and health education has been used. This included developing and enforcing the use seat belts, special car seats for smaller children, motorcycle and bicycle helmets with face-guards, as well as enforcing speed limit for motor vehicles. Also, the development of bicycle lanes and zebra cross for pedestrians. This was followed by health education to developing an awareness of traffic hazards and the benefits of using engineering protective devices, and to improve road safety behaviour and skills. This may explain the small proportion of traffic related traumatic dental injuries (??%) observed in East London (Marcenes and Murray, in press). Therefore, it seems possible to reduce the prevalence of traumatic dental injuries if traffic and other health promotion strategies related to physical leisure activities and violence is implemented.

Physical leisure activities related health promotion strategies

The other major event related to traumatic dental injury is physical leisure activities. Dental health professionals can provide well-fitting mouth guards to children to use when playing sports. Dental health professionals may pressure for legislation to enforce the use of protective devices when engaging in risky physical activities. Health education should focus on increasing awareness of the risk of engaging in physical activities without adequate protection, for example, rollerblading without protective devices. Health education should also stress the benefits of formal training and improving fitness before engaging in risky leisure physical activities.

Violence related health promotion strategies

Another major event related to traumatic dental injury is violence. Since traumatic dental injuries may be due to physical abuse including bullying from peers, dental health professionals should be able to identify and act against violence. It is important that dental health professionals start to recognising the signs and symptoms of physical abuse, developing office policies and procedures for documenting and reporting suspected cases, and collaborating with other community members to help preventing violence. This may also save lives. Data from the UK showed that 4 children die each day through non-accidental injury or neglect, 4.2 out of a 1,000 children have been physically abused; and that 5% of children who has been physically abused dies and 35% are seriously re-injured if returned without protective intervention. Despite its seriousness few health professionals are prepared to report suspicious cases of child abuse.

A case for the common risk factor approach

Because unintentional and intentional harmful events are the main causes of traumatic dental injuries and other body injuries, a common risk factor approach should be adopted and the prevention of TDI should be incorporated into general health promotion strategies designed to prevent other type of injuries. In addition, the prevention of TDI offers a great opportunity to dental health professionals to collaborate with other health professionals and to contribute to solve a serious public health problem. Injuries are responsible for 7% of world mortality, are the leading cause of death in children older than 1 year and account for 15% of all healthy years of life lost. In addition, non-fatal injuries cause significant disability and have a very high cost to society.

Prevention of the outcome of traumatic dental injuries

It is important to stress that to provide treatment for traumatic dental injuries is an important health promotion strategy. The treatment of traumatic dental injuries is an important health promotion strategy that may prevent significant biological and social negative impacts. Dental treatment may restore the ability of enjoying food, tooth cleaning, smiling and showing teeth without embarrassment, maintaining an emotional state without being irritable, and socialising.

Optimal care should include first aid, pre-hospital care, out-of-hours services and in-hours services.

Oral health professionals should teach the public, in particular parents and school teachers, who are likely to be close to the injured person at the time of the harmful

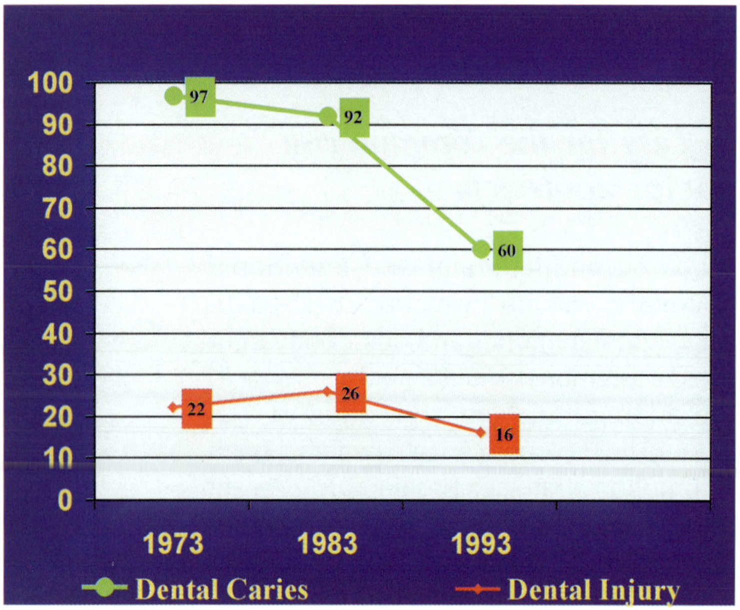

Fig. 3.2 Trends in caries and traumatised teeth in 15 years old english children.

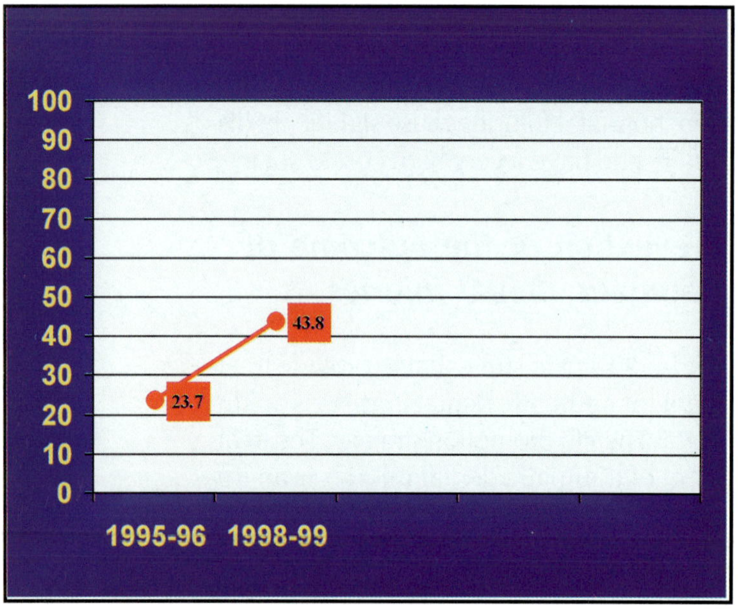

Fig. 3.3 Prevalence of traumatised teeth in 14 years old children in Newham, London in 1995-96 and 1998-99 (Marcenes e Murray, 2002).

event, the correct management of damaged teeth. This is because the immediate care of damaged teeth is crucial for a successful outcome of treatment. Out-of-hour services are very important too and must be provided because most of traumatic dental injuries events happened out of working hours. High quality treatment should be provided to prevent bacterial invasion in the exposed dentinal tubules leading to inflammation that could lead to necrosis of the pulp, as well as to assure children the capacity to perform desired social roles.

References

1. Andreasen JO, Andreasen FM. *Textbook and color atlas of traumatic injuries to the teeth.* 3. ed. Copenhagen: Munksgaard; 1994.
2. Andreasen JO, Ravn JJ. Epidemiology of traumatic dental injuries to primary and permanent teeth in a Danish population sample. *Int J Oral Surg,* 1972; 1:235-9.
3. Borssen A, Holm AK. Traumatic dental injuries in a cohort of 16-year-olds in Northen Sweden. *Endod Dent Traumatol,* 1997;13:276-80.
4. Bigela, MFTB. Estudo de traumatismo em incisivos permanentes de escolares brasileiros de Bauru. Estado de São Paulo, Tese de Doutorado, USP, 1972.
5. Brown, L. Research in dental health education and health promotion: a review of the literature. *Health Education Quarterly,* 1994, 21, 83-102.
6. Cortes MIS, Marcenes W, Sheiham A. Prevalence and correlates of traumatic injuries to the permanent teeth of schoolchildren aged 9-14 years in Belo Horizonte, Brazil. *Endod Dent Traumatol* 2001;17:22-26.
7. Cortes MIS, Marcenes W, Sheiham A. The impact of traumatic injuries to the permanent teeth on oral health related quality of life of 12 to 14 year old Brazilian school-children. *Community Dent Oral Epidemiol,* 2001, 30: 193-8.
8. Editorial. The Melburne Declaration. *Injury Prevention,* 1996; 2, 83.
9. Golder M. Non-Acident Injury in Children. Dent Update, 1995; 22:75 80.
10. Hamilton FA, Hill FJ, Holloway PJ. An investigation of dento-alveolar trauma and its treatment in an adolescent population. Part 1: The prevalence and incidence of injuries and the extent and adequacy of treatment received. *Br Dent J,* 1997;182, 91-5.
11. Huang BY, Marcenes W, Croucher RE, Hector, MP. Accidental and non-accidental causes of injuries to teeth: a critical literature review. Final programme and abstracts – 18th Congress of the International Association of Pediatric Dentistry, Paris 2001. Abstract TP3-14, p 51.
12. Kay L, Locker D. Effectiveness of oral health promotion. Health Education Authority, Health Promotion Effectiveness reviews.
13. Kay L, Locker D. Is dental health education effective? A systematic review of current evidence. *Community Dent Oral Epidemiol,* 1996; 24, 231-5.
14. Marcenes W, Alessi ON, Traebert J. Causes and prevalence of traumatic injuries to the permanent incisors of schoolchildren aged 12 years in Jaragua do Sul, Brazil. *Int Dent J*; 2000; 50:87-92.
15. Marcenes W; Murray S. Changes in Prevalence and Treatment Need for Traumatic Dental Injuries Among 14 year-old Children in Newham, London: A Depreved Area. *Community Dent Health,* 2002;19:104-108.
16. Marcenes W, Murray S. Social deprivation and traumatic dental injuries among 14 -year-old schoolchildren in Newham, London. *Endod Dent Traumatol,* 2000; 16; 1-5.
17. Marcenes W, Murray S. Deprivation, changes in prevalence and treatment needed due to traumatic dental injuries among 14-year-old children in Newham, London: a deprived area. *Community Dent Health,* 2002; 19: 104-8.
18. Marcenes W, Zabot NE, Traebert J. Socio-economic correlates of traumatic injuries to the permanent incisors in schoolchildren aged 12 years in Blumenau, Brazil. *Endod Dental Traumatol*; 2001; 17:222-226.
19. Nicolau B, Marcenes W, Sheiham A. Prevalence, causes and correlates of traumatic dental injuries among 13 years olds in Brazil. *Endod Dent Traumatol*; 2001;17:213-217.
20. O'Brien M. Children's Dental health in the United Kingdom 1993. In: *Report of Dental Survey, Office of Population Censuses and Surveys.* London: Her Majesty's Stationery Office; 1994.
21. Schou L, Locker D. Oral health: a review of the effectiveness of health education and health promotion. Dutch Centre for Health Promotion and Health Education, 1994.
22. Shanger RG; Bross DC. Implications of Child Abuse and Negueched for the

Dental Profession. *J Am Dent Assoc,* 1982;104:55-56.

23. Sprod A, Anderson R, Treasure E. Effective oral health promotion. Literature Review. Health Promotion Wales, 1996.
24. Traebert J, Almeida ICS, Garghetti C and Marcenes W (no prelo). Prevalência, necessidade de tratamento e fatores predisponentes do traumatismo dentário na dentição permanente de escolares de 11 a 13 anos de idade. *Cadernos de Saúde Pública.*

Chapter **4**

Malocclusion in a Public Health Context

Cesar Messias de Oliveira

Introduction

Two centuries ago, the famous English poet William Cowper stated, "Variety's the very spice of life, that gives it all its flavour". To paraphrase Cowper, occlusal variation is the real spice of the orthodontic treatment specialty that gives it all its flavour.

The assessment of occlusion for public health purposes has two main objectives. The first is to screen the population for individual treatment need and priority. The second is to obtain information for planning, resources and facilities for orthodontic treatment.[1]

Epidemiologists also need a method for the accurate assessment of occlusal variations to increase scientific knowledge about occlusion and to study the relationship of the various occlusal traits or combinations of traits to different characteristics in a population.

Although epidemiological studies of malocclusion have been reported in various countries, comparison is difficult. The indices and criteria used are not standardized. Methods for an objective evaluation of dental caries and periodontal disease are established, but similar methods for malocclusion have yet to be defined. At present, even the Global Oral Data Bank of the World Health Organization has only limited data concerning malocclusion.

During the last decades there has been an increasing demand for orthodontic treatment, which may be for a number of reasons namely, the general improvement in the oral health of children with a decline in caries; increased dental awareness and expectations; and increased availability of care. As a result of this increased demand, waiting lists and waiting times for orthodontic treatment have grown. In the UK, where the General Dental Service, the Community Dental Service, and the Hospital Dental Service provide orthodontic treatment, there is an uneven regional uptake for treatment, which is strongly related to the distributions of orthodontic manpower.

In response to the increased pressures indices have been developed which attempt to prioritise patients in accordance with the severity of their malocclusions and treatment need. Researchers have used these indices in order to assess the orthodontic treatment need in different populations.

The provision of orthodontic services in publicly funded programmes is becoming a concern with increased number of orthodontic treatment demand on the one hand, and limited resources and manpower on the other.

It is important; therefore, to make sure that the methodology used to assess malocclusions and orthodontic treatment need in relation to accessing public health programmes is valid.

The assessment of malocclusion and treatment need for public health purposes is necessary for the following reasons: firstly, to help determine priorities of access for services provision under publicly-funded programmes; secondly, to estimate the need for treatment in a population with respect to training an adequate number of providers; and finally, for planning resources and facilities to meet both actual and potential demand for such treatment.

However, many problems exist in estimating need for orthodontic treatment in a public health context. Different examiners, carrying out surveys in different areas, have found a wide variation in the proportion of subjects recommended for treatment. This wide variation reflects a lack of uniform standards for defining deviations from ideal occlusion severe enough to need orthodontic treatment. Recent research findings have indicated that the main benefit of orthodontic treatment to the patient may be in improved dental aesthetics and psychosocial well-being.[2] Consequently, recent developments in the assessment of orthodontic treatment need attempts to measure the aesthetic impairment and psychosocial need.

Surveys carried out in the UK have expressed doubts about the 'validity' of the orthodontic indices used, i.e. the extent to which the index measures what it purports to measure.[3] Even today there is insufficient reliable data on the functional and psychosocial impacts of malocclusion to permit true scientific validation of indices of orthodontic treatment need. However, because IOTN has been developed using all the currently available scientific data and concurs with a broad consensus of professional opinions in the UK, it represents an important advance in the evolution of orthodontic indices. Additionally, as only the most severe occlusal trait is recorded, the IOTN index is a quick and reliable method when used to assess treatment needs at a community level.

Thus, researchers involved in developing measures of orthodontic treatment need have been hampered by a shortage of data on the detrimental effects of malocclusion,[4-6] and difficulties in quantifying the social and psychological impact of malocclusion. Despite these constraints the recently developed Index of Orthodontic Treatment Need[7] is gaining widespread acceptance by clinicians in the UK.

The aim of the present chapter is to discuss the epidemiology of malocclusion and its public health aspects. This chapter will provide an overview about the assessment of malocclusion throughout the world and, mainly, the development of occlusal indices particularly, the Index of Orthodontic Treatment Need (IOTN). In addition, it will review the literature relating to the impacts of malocclusion.

Epidemiology of malocclusion

In order to assess whether malocclusion is considered to be a public health problem, the prevalence of occlusal anomalies, the need and demand for orthodontic treatment should be ascertained within a given community.[8] This would help identify appropriate arrangements for the allocation of resources.[9,10]

Epidemiological studies of the prevalence of malocclusion in populations date back to the early 1900s. In 1899, Angle first established his classification of occlusion based on molar relationship that is still used today. His sample of 1000 Caucasians showed 69% to have normal occlusion or Class I malocclusion, 23% class II, 3.4% class III malocclusions, and the remaining 4.6% had asymmetric occlusions. Chiavaro,[11] Korkhans[12] and Hill et al.[13] published surveys showing general agreement with the findings of Angle's study on the distribution of malocclusions.

Most studies in their attempt to determine the prevalence of malocclusion have divided malocclusion into five components:

- crowding;
- anteroposterior incisor relation (overjet/ reverse overjet);
- anteroposterior molar relationship;
- incisor relationship and
- crossbite relationship.

Epidemiological studies of malocclusions have been documented in Europe and North America using established epidemiological indices (Table 1). The few studies on the prevalence of malocclusion reported in Africa are difficult to compare because of the diversity of recording methods used (Table 2). The prevalence of class I cases (normal and malocclusion) in Africa is about 80%. The frequency of class II malocclusion seems to vary from 18% in Libya[14] to 1.3% in South Africa.[15] The class II cases in African children are less frequent than those reported in other parts of the world. A high prevalence of class III malocclusion was found in many different countries in Africa.

According to Isiekwe[27] the high incidence of decreased overjet is undoubtedly associated with the low prevalence of class II and the high incidence of bimaxillary proclination. Crowding in the maxillary and mandibular anterior segments was seen in 6.0% and 5.0% respectively in the Sudan.[28] Richardson and Ana[29] in a Nigerian sample found crowding in 18.0% in the maxilla and

Table 4.1 Prevalence of malocclusion in Europe and North America.

Author/year	Country	Sample	Age	Normal occlusion	Class I (%)	Class II (%)	Class III (%)
Sclare (1945)[16]	England	334	12	40.5	30.0	27.0	1.0
Bjork (1947)[17]	Sweden	322	12	26.4	51.8	18.9	2.8
Massler e Frankel (1951)[18]	USA	2.758	14-18	21.1	50.0	20.0	9.0
Telle (1951)[19]	Norway	2.349	7-8	41.3	30.1	21.3	7.3
Gardiner (1956)[20]	England	1.000	6-15	25.0	66.0	8.2	1.0
Goose et al. (1957)[21]	England	953	11-12	55.3	25.0	15.7	2.7
Altemus (1959)[22]	USA	537	12	17.0	63.6	14.4	4.6
Hill et al. (1959)[13]	USA	1.888	12-14	52.6	33.5	12.7	1.1
Breham e Jackson (1961)[23]	USA	6.328	6-17	16.6	60.1	22.8	0.5
Haynes (1970)[24]	England	1.185	11-12	26.8	50.3	19.5	2.5
Foster e Walpole (1974)[25]	England	1.000	11-12	–	44.3	52.2	3.5
Robert e Goose (1979)[26]	England	100	12	–	62.0	28.0	9.0

Table 4.2 Prevalence of malocclusion in different Arab, African and South American countries.

Author/year	Country	Sample size	Age	Class I (%)	Class II (%)	Class III (%)
Arab countries						
Lundstrom e Lundstrom (1969)[35]	Egypt	318	6-18	60.0	7.0	4.0
Gardiner (1982)[14]	Libya	500	10-12	77.0	18.0	5.0
Nashashibi et al. (1983)[36]	Saudi Arabia	1.000	9-14	85.2 (f)	9.0 (f)	5.6 (f)
			75.2 (m)	19.0 (m)	5.6 (m)	
Steigman et al. (1983)[37]	Israel	803	13-15	85.3	10.0	1.3
Farawana (1987)[38]	Iraq	200	6-24	59.6	29.6	10.8
African countries						
Jacobson (1967)[39]	South Africa	460	Adults	97.4 (f)	2.6 (f)	(f) –
			96,4 (m)	2.9 (m)	0.7 (m)	
Richardson & Ana (1973)[29]	Nigeria	100	6-7	80.0 (f)	8.0 (f)	16.0 (f)
			84.0 (m)	8.0 (m)	16.0 (m)	
		100	13-14	82.0 (f)	8.0 (f)	8.0 (f)
			76.0 (m)	10.0 (m)	12.0 (m)	
		100	18-22	86.0 (f)	8.0 (f)	18.0 (f)
			76.0 (m)	8.0 (m)	14.0 (m)	
Hirschowitz et al. (1981)[15]	South Africa	402	12	98.0	1.0	1.0
Isiekwe (1982)[27]	Nigeria	617	10-19	76.8	14.7	8.4
Kapila (1983)[40]	Kenya	686	2-20	85.0	2.3	13.0
Garner e Butt (1985)[41]	Kenya	505	13-15	68.5	7.9	16.8
Diagne et al. (1988)[43]	Senegal	1.708	11-19	73.3	12.7	4.4
Kerusuo et al. (1988)[43]	Tanzania	642	11-13	96	3	1
South American Countries						
Silva Filho et al. (1990)[31]	Brazil	2.416	7-11	55	42	3
Muniz (1986)[30]	Argentina	1.554	12-13	85	10	5

(f) = Female **(m) = Male** **– = No record**

24.0% in the mandible. Prevalence of spacing in the anterior-segments was quite high in Africa: Sudan, 18.0% and Libya, 20%. The occurrence of midline diastema is considered a sign of natural beauty in Senegal, Sudan, Nigeria, Tanzania and Kenya.

In Latin America, there are also very few nation-wide epidemiological studies on the prevalence of malocclusion (Table 4.2). Furthermore, they are difficult to compare because of the diversity of evaluation criteria used. For example, Muniz[30] assessed malocclusion traits in Argentine children aged 12-13 using the WHO – FDI basic method for recording occlusal traits. The frequency of distal molar relation was 10% and the mesial molar relation 5%. In Brazil, Silva Filho et al.[31] using the Angle's classification, found class I malocclusions the most prevalent (55%), followed by class II (42%) and, finally, by class III (3%).

Some studies in the literature report the

Table 4.3 Occlusal variation among different ethnic groups.

Author/year	Nationality	Sample size	Age	Malocclusion	Class I (%)	Class II (%)	Class III (%)
Baume (1974)[33]	Polynesian	19.854	3-60	[a]	[a]	10.0	5.5
El-Mangoury e Mostafa (1990)[32]	Egyptian	501	18-24	65.7[b]	33.3	21.0	10.6
Garner e Butt (1985)[41]	Black american	445	13-15	73.0[b]	44.0	16.0	8.7
Garner e Butt (1985)[41]	Kikuyu kenyan	505	13-14	83.2[b]	51.7	7.9	16.8
Goose et al. (1957)[21]	British	2.956	7-15	32.7	13.7	16.1	2.9
Grewe et al. (1968)[44]	Indian	651	9-14	65.5	53.0	9.6	2.9
Helm (1968)[34]	Danish	3.842	6-18	78.5	49.7	24.5	4.3
Horowitz (1970)[45]	American	718	10-12	93.2	65.2	22.5	5.5
Ingervall (1974)46	Swedish	301[c]	18[d]	90.0	83.0	3.0	4.0
Laine e Hausen (1983)[47]	Finnish	451	17-51	[a]	[a]	15.0	5.0
Salzmann (1977)[48]	American	7.514	12-17	100.00[e]	54.0	32.0	14.0
Siriwat e Jarabak (1985)[49]	American	500	8-12	100.00[e]	47.2	46.4	6.4
Solow e Helm (1968)[50]	Danish	275	[f]	72.8	37.4	34.0	1.4
Wood (1971)[51]	Eskimo	100	11-20	82.0	64.0	8.0	10.0

[a] No figures reported
[b] Malocclusion prevalence including Angle Class IV
[c] Male sample
[d] Only mean age reported (age range not reported)
[e] Malocclusion sample only
[f] Children

prevalence of Angle's malocclusion types in terms of different ethnic groups, (Table 3). Occlusal variation differs numerically among different world populations. These differences could be attributed to a number of factors. However, the occlusal variation follows a universal general distribution pattern for most world populations. Specifically, this pattern is arranged in the following descending order: Angle class I, Angle class II, and Angle class III[32]. The exception to this trend is noted in Chinese, Malays and, to a lesser extent, Eskimos and Swedes. Although some of these differences in incidences reflect ethnic trends, a host of other factors also contribute to these variations. Some of these include differences in age[33], sex[25] and definition of evaluation criteria and the lack of standardisation amongst examiners.

Helm[34] believes that a considerable proportion of the variability in the frequencies of malocclusion obtained by different research workers is due to differences in subjective criteria for the recorded items, rather than reflecting inherent differences between the various population groups. If reliable estimates of the prevalence of malocclusion have been difficult to establish, then the reported incidence of orthodontic treatment needs is even more contentious.

Table 4.4. Prevalence of common occlusal anomalies (%).

Intra-arch traits	(%)	Interarch traits	(%)
Hypodontia		**Overjet**	
Permanent teeth (except			
third molars)	6	< 0	3
Upper lateral incisors	1-2	+ ve < 5 mm	76
Premolars	1	5-7 mm	14
	> 7 mm	8	
Hyperdontia			
Supernumary teeth	0,1-4	**Overbite**	
		> 5 mm incisal coverage	11-24
Ectopic eruption		> 7 mm incisal coverage	3
One or more 16, 26	4	Traumatic	1
One or more 13, 23	2	Open bite	2-4
		Dentoalveolar disproportion	
Infraocclusion, deciduous molars	14	Deciduous	
		Spacing (age)	90-95
Cross-bite		Permanent	
Posterior		Spacing > 2 mm	9
Unilateral	10		
Bilateral	2	**Crowding**	
Anterior	7	> 2 mm	16-26
With displacement	75	> 3 mm	25
Lingual	7-8	> 6 mm	7
	> 9 mm	3	
Median diastema			
Before eruption 12, 22	95	**Miscellaneous**	
After eruption 12, 22	25	Digit/dummy sucking	
	Age: 3 years	42	
	Age: 12 years	7	

Estimates of the frequency of different traits of malocclusion are available from a number of different surveys, mainly north European and north American. Direct comparison between surveys is not generally possible as estimates vary according to the examining criteria adopted, levels of severity, sampling differences of age and gender, availability of study casts and radiographs (for detecting unerupted teeth), and the accuracy of the examiners. A brief synopsis of a number of surveys is presented in table 4.4.

From a review of the literature, it appears that reliable estimates of the prevalence of malocclusion have been difficult to establish. This has probably been due to the fact that most classifications and studies on the epidemiology of malocclusion have been qualitative in nature and subjective in method. The most commonly used qualitative assessment of malocclusion is the Angle[57] classification of malocclusion.

Assessing orthodontic treatment need

One of the major problems in orthodontic diagnosis and assessment of orthodontic treatment need, is that orthodontic anomaly is not a disease with a series of well-recognised symptoms. It is a variation from the norm in which treatment is based upon the evaluation of certain dental characteristics in an otherwise healthy person. Orthodontic treatment need is difficult to define precisely because of the uncertainty of the functional and psychological benefits of orthodontic treatment[53]. It is often the perception of the professional that is used to define the dental treatment. Orthodontics is the field of dentistry with the most contested concepts because deviations from the 'normal' occlusion are not clear-cut unless one adopts a very strict normative approach, where any misalignment should be treated.

Classic orthodontic teaching has emphasised that the major benefits of orthodontic treatment are the improvement of physical function, the prevention of tissue destruction and the correction of aesthetic impairment[54]. A re-evaluation of the benefits of orthodontic treatment is currently taking place as a result of recent research findings.[55-58] Contemporary orthodontic opinion is beginning to doubt the importance of orthodontic care for prevention of caries, periodontal disease and temporomandibular disorders.[59] According to orthodontist Isaacson,[60] "... orthodontic care appears to be unjustifiable on the basis that without it negative sequelae will occur." Prahl-Andersen[61] questions the traditional assumptions underlying the need for orthodontic treatment. She claims that the belief that individuals with 'ideal' occlusion have significantly fewer caries, less periodontal disease and function better than individuals with malocclusion, has not been clearly demonstrated.

In his thesis, 'Reappraisal of the criteria for orthodontic treatment', Helm[62] stated that "the assessment of need or indication for treatment can indeed be the orthodontist's most difficult task". On the basis of the research findings he concluded that most malocclusions have a smaller impact on oral health (e.g. caries, periodontal disease) than previously anticipated. On the other hand, the hypothesis that malocclusions did create psychosocial problems, which are not necessarily easier to cope with than somatic problems, was confirmed. Current research provides less support than previously believed for the physical benefits derived from the provision of orthodontic treatment of malocclusio.[55-58] Although severe malocclusion may compromise some aspects of oral function, Proffit[63] believes that less severe malocclusion will not compromise function, but may still require some physiological compensation.

This review of need for orthodontic treatment will not deal with all the assumptions of orthodontists of what comprise a malocclusion. Instead, the main indications for treatment will be discussed. Two diverse viewpoints by influential professors of orthodontics illustrate the range of indications. On the one hand, Shaw et al.[53] states that there is evidence that more severe dental features such as traumatic deep overbite, unprotected incisors and impacted teeth adversely affect the longevity of the dentition. He also stated that the relationship of dental irregularity to periodontal disease, caries and mandibular dysfunction is less certain. At the other extreme, Solow[64] developed a list of indications for intervention for orthodontic treatment, which is not evidence based (Table 4.5).

Solow's indications for orthodontic treatment are currently used in Denmark. The difference in approach between Shaw and Solow demonstrates why the prevalence of children needing orthodontic treatment varies so greatly, both within countries and between examiners. In 10 industrialised countries a range of between 21% and 64% of 13 to 14 year olds were reported to 'need' orthodontic treatment.[65] Although some differences are to be expected in the prevalence of orthodontic treatment need, it is likely that this large variation in need reflects the inherent subjectivity of the evaluation systems used[66] and their questionable validity and reliability.[3]

Table 4.5. Health risks related to malocclusion.[64]

Risk	Malocclusion
I Risk of damage to the teeth and surrounding tissue	
1. Caries	Rarely justifies orthodontic treatment
2. Periodontal lesions	Extreme deep bite Pronounced anterior cross-bite or reverse overjet Pronounced crowding
3. Traumatic dental injuries	Extreme overjet, particularly when the teeth are not protected by the lips
4. Extreme wear of the teeth	Forced biteDeep bite with retroclined upper incisors
5. Root resorption of the upper incisors	Unerupted ectopic upper canines
II Risk of functional disorders	
1. Cranio-mandibular disorders	Forced bite (forwards, backwards, laterally) Lack of occlusal stability
2. Chewing and/or incising difficulties	Pronounced anterior or lateral open bite Pronounced reverse overjet Locking of the bite due to extensive lingual or buccal crossbite Pronounced anterior cross-bite
3. Speech disorders	Rarely justify orthodontic treatment
III Risk of psychosocial stress	
Teasing, harassment, low self-esteem	Facial deformities, cleft lip Extreme overjet Reverse overjet Pronounced crowding, particularly of the upper incisors and canines Pronounced spacing of the upper incisors
IV Risk of late sequelae	
1. Forward migration of the upper incisors	Extreme overjet with lip trapping incisors
2. Late development of extreme deep bite	Extreme jaw growth in connection with lack of incisal contact
3. Asymmetric facial development	Pronounced lateral lingual or buccal cross-bite with forced bite

In some Scandinavian countries the percentage of children having orthodontic treatment is about 35%. However, because of cost pressures, orthodontists in Denmark are expected to reduce the percentage of children having orthodontics to 25%.[64] As a consequence decisions will have to be made on who will benefit most and indications for intervention will have to change. Perhaps the indications for intervention outlined by Salzmann,[67] who defined a handicapping malocclusion, as one that adversely affects aesthetics, function or speech, is more relevant than the predominantly clinical indications recommended by Solow.[64] The definition of the aims of the orthodontic treatment of the British Dental Association[68] captures some of the emphasis of psychosocial aspects of teeth: "to produce improved function by the correction of irregularities and to create not only greater resistance to disease, but also to improve personal appearance, which later will contribute to the mental as well as to the physical well-being of the individual". A similar emphasis was expressed by the World Health Organization.[65] Malocclusion is considered a handicapping dentofacial anomaly and defined as an anomaly, which causes disfigurement or impedes function, and requires treatment "if the disfigurement or functional defect is, or is likely to be, an obstacle to the patient's physical or emotional well-being".

Prahl-Andersen[61] discussed the concept of treatment need from the point of view of three types of information collected in the practice of medicine. These were objective signs, subjective symptoms, and social sufficiency. Objective signs involve those anomalies that deviate sufficiently from the recognised norm, while subjective symptoms refer to self-perception of the presence of an anomaly that is in need of treatment. Social sufficiency considers the recognition by society that the individual's malocclusion is in need of treatment, and this is related to current sociocultural norms for appearance.

Shaw et al.[4-6] showed that the criteria used by dentists to judge need for orthodontic treatment are not clear and there is ample scope for subjective assessment. Accordingly, it is difficult to see how the assessment of treatment need, and by inference, outcomes of treatment, could be completely objective. Nevertheless, the overemphasis on clinical measures and the imprecise and often casual assessment of the psychosocial aspects needs readdressing.

The issue of how orthodontic diagnostic and treatment decisions are made and outcomes of treatment are measured, has considerable interest in a future of technology transfer where medical algorithms have been devised for the diagnosis and treatment of disease. The shifting paradigm in orthodontics will not be centred on growth prediction, with orthodontists' intent on modifying and redirect craniofacial growth, but will focus future efforts on those aspects of treatment where the orthodontist has some direct control by making evidence-based diagnostic and treatment decisions.[69]

It is not merely the elective nature of orthodontic treatment that makes it unique. It is also the way in which it differs from medicine by virtue of the outcome measures on which assessments of costs, risks and benefits of treatment are based. An important but undressed question for orthodontists is whether society or the individual should pay for orthodontic care. Clinical trials in medicine can, and usually do, estimate outcomes of tangible benefit to patients.[70]

The range of concepts relating to estimating needs for orthodontic treatment also applies to the assessment of the outcomes of orthodontic care.

Occlusal indices

In recent years there has been an increased interest in the development of methods to reduce subjectivity in the assessment of both treatment needs and treatment standards. To this end, various indices have been developed in dentistry to provide objective measurements. In orthodontics this role may be fulfilled by the use of occlusal indices that record traits of malocclusion in numerical or categorical format, in order to maximise objectivity and minimise subjectivity. There have been many attempts to produce a malocclusion index that could be used to record incidence, prevalence, and treatment need of malocclusion (Table 4.6).

Occlusal indices may be defined as methods of determining the level of treatment need or the amount of deviation from a normal occlusion. They can be used both for the evaluation of individual patients and populations and as indicators of the clinical outcome of orthodontic treatment. Eco-

Table 4.6. Summary of methods for recording malocclusion.

Author(s) and Year of Development	Nature of Method
Angle (1899)[52]	Qualitative
Stallard (1932)[71]	Qualitative
McCall (1944)[72]	Qualitative
Sclare (1945)[16]	Qualitative
Massler & Frankel (1951)[18]	Quantitative
Vankirk & Pennell (1959)[73]	Quantitative
Draker (1960)[8]	Quantitative
Fisk (1960)[74]	Qualitative
Grainger (1960)[75]	Quantitative
Poulton & Aaronson (1961)[76]	Quantitative
Bjork et al. (1964)[77]	Qualitative
Summers (1971)[78]	Quantitative
Grainger (1967)[79]	Quantitative
Salzmann (1968)[67]	Quantitative
Profitt & Ackerman (1973)[80]	Qualitative
Linder-Aronson (1974)[81]	Grade Index Scale
Brzroukov et al. (1979)[82]	Qualitative
Kinaar & Burke (1981)[83]	Qualitative
Cons et al. (1986)[84]	Quantitative
Brook & Shaw (1989)[7]	Grade Index Scale
Daniels & Richmond (2000)[85]	Quantitative

nomic restraints in recent years have resulted in an increasing interest in the evaluation of orthodontic treatment outcome. Occlusal indices have been used to assess outcome for orthodontic treatment and need, the following is a critical review of the literature.

It is a basic requirement of any index or system of measurement, that it should be valid and reproducible. Validity is the ability of an index to measure that which it purports to measure, whereas reproducibility is the ability to reproduce the original ratings or scores when the subject is reexamined by the same or a different examiner. A good index should be easy to learn, ideally allowing rapid recording of relevant features by both trained dental and nondental personnel.[86]

For most of this century, the dental profession has directed considerable attention to methods of description and measurement of malocclusion. The apparent lack of universally accepted measuring techniques for assessing need and outcomes for orthodontic treatment derives to a large extent from the inherent complexities of the underlying basic science of craniofacial growth and development. In addition, aetiology of malocclusion, orthodontic diagnosis, and effects of malocclusion are by nature multi-factorial.[87] Orthodontic patients have different growth patterns, psychological and cultural needs. Below, some general trends in which the orthodontic profession has described and measured malocclusion during the last century will be briefly reviewed.

Although some classification systems for systematic description of observations were suggested in the 19th century, none were generally accepted until Edward Angle[52] introduced the concept 'malocclusion' and established a simple system by dividing malocclusions into three main types. Despite criticism and many shortcomings, Angle's typological classification has so far become the only universally acknowledged method still in regular use. The method was devised as an attempt to systematise treatment planning, and has served as a tool for professional communication. However, the method has frequently been used for other purposes, and often been applied in epidemiological studies.

One purpose of epidemiological studies of malocclusion is to provide data for organising care. Analysis of the adverse effects of malocclusion and the identification of etiologic factors depends upon detailed measurements of the various malocclusion traits that are not included in typological classifications. In response to the need for more sophisticated tools, methods for recording all the single traits of a malocclusion were developed. One example of this approach is the method established by Bjork, Krebs and Solow[77] by which definitions and criteria for all single traits that constitute a person's malocclusion were defined. In addition to studying the prevalence of traits, this methodology is suitable for analysing associations between malocclusion and dental factors such as caries, periodontal disease and function.

Another approach is to measure deviations from the norm by assigning scores to various occlusal traits that are then added to obtain a total score. Several indices based on a summary score have been devised and used to assess prevalence of malocclusion. The advantage of indices which express malocclusion by a summary score is that a person's occlusal status can be considered as a quantitative variable. A disadvantage is that different malocclusions may result in the same score. A scoring procedure that measures malocclusion quantitatively may be most suitable for the general evaluation of treatment outcome in terms of improvement in occlusion. The PAR-Index recently developed in Great Britain[88] is designed specifically to assess changes in occlusion as a result of treatment.

In response to the development of programs for the organization and funding of orthodontic care, starting in the middle of this century, a number of indices were proposed with the intention of identifying individuals with a need for treatment.[8,78,79,89] The recognition that measuring severity of malocclusion in terms of the degree of deviation was not equivalent to determining the need for treatment, lead to the development of indices that apply weightings. Values have been given to scores depending on the location of the deviation in the dental arch, or on the degree of the deviation. It has been recognised that treatment priority indices designed to objectively interpret the severity of malocclusions, nevertheless commonly use index scores that are based on clinical estimates.[90,91] Even if weighting procedures have been based on multiple regression models, or validated by applying professional assessment panels, clinical judgement remains the underlying principle.

During the 1960's and 1970's it gradually became apparent that the measurement of orthodontic treatment need was compounded by the variation in professional and patient perception of what constitutes a malocclusion.[61] Barmes[92] in a review of attempts made by the WHO[93,94] to define dentofacial anomalies stated that the usefulness of orthodontic indices has been severely limited by a failure to devise a precise definition of an anomaly and of when it requires treatment. The problem can mainly be attributed to the variability in perception, not only by the potential patient, but also by the dental specialist, general practitioner or epidemiologist.

To reconcile professional and patient perceptions, Barmes[92] recommended to first define several levels of need for various populations. These levels should then be modified in terms of patient perceptions as an essential final step. The clinical definitions of the level of need should be re-evaluated by an assessment of the number of people at various levels who, on the basis of individual perception, would be placed in a different category. It would take adequate samples at each level of clinical definition of need to quantify the differences between patient and professional assessments.

In conclusion, the indices of orthodontic treatment need consist of a metric specification of how irregular the malocclusion is or how great the deviation is from the 'ideal' occlusion. In other words, they are based on an idea that the greater the deviation from the 'ideal' occlusion is, the greater the risks of oral health problems are. Such indices of orthodontic treatment need do not take into account the psychosocial aspects of malocclusion.

Recent developments of indices of orthodontic treatment need

Presently, there is no comprehensive measure of outcome for orthodontic treatment. Assuming that treatment reduces need and consequently contributes to health gain, it would be prudent to review recent developments of assessing orthodontic need. The recent indices of orthodontic treatment need will be considered using the criteria outlined by Sheiham and Spencer[95] namely that there should be:

- a clinical dimension based upon sound concepts of the life history of the condition, in this case growth and development;
- a measure which incorporates functional measures of the impacts of impairment;
- measures of social dysfunction;
- a measure to evaluate the wants of the individual;
- a measure of the propensity of the individual to adhere to the treatment regimen and the perceived barriers and
- a prescription of effective and acceptable treatments and the professional skills required to carry them out.

Over the past two decades an increasing number of studies on lay persons' attitudes to dentofacial anomalies have been published.[62,96-98] Concurrently, indices establishing categories of orthodontic treatment need have been in operation in the Scandinavian countries whilst indices defining levels of treatment need have been utilised in the United Kingdom. Surprisingly, few orthodontic treatment need indices have attempted to measure or record the perceptions of the child or parent in relation to psychosocial aspects of malocclusion. One index, the Index of Orthodontic Treatment Need (IOTN), was developed in the United Kingdom and ranks malocclusion in terms of the significance of various occlusal traits for the individual's dental health and perceived aesthetic impairment. The intention of identifying those individuals is to establish who would be most likely to benefit from orthodontic treatment. The index incorporates a dental health and an aesthetic component.[7]

The dental health component of the IOTN represents an attempt at synthesis of the current evidence for the deleterious effects of malocclusion and the potential benefits of orthodontic treatment, loosely based upon the Index of the Swedish Medical Board. Each occlusal trait thought to contribute to the longevity and satisfactory functioning of the dentition is defined and placed into five grades, with clear cut-off points between the grades. Grade 1 represents a negligible need for treatment while grade 5 indicates an urgent or high priority for treatment. Ten features or traits of malocclusion are used to establish the grade level. These are overjet, overbite, openbite, crossbite, displacement of teeth, impeded eruption of teeth, defects of cleft lip and palate, class II and class II buccal occlusions, and hypodontia. These various features of the malocclusion are noted and measured, with a specially designed ruler. A fundamental premise of the index is the recognition that dental conditions are site-specific (for example, severe displacement of a particular tooth represents a particular disadvantage for that site). The most severe trait identified is the basis for grading the individual's need for orthodontic treatment on dental health grounds. Summing scores for a series of individual traits is not performed. Thus, multiple minor variations, which are unimportant with respect to dental health, cannot be added together to place an individual in a higher grade (Box 4.1).

The aesthetic component of the IOTN consists of a 10-point scale, illustrated by a series of numbered photographs which were rated for attractiveness by lay individuals and selected as being equidistantly spaced through the range of scores (Fig. 4.1). This aesthetic component can be ranked by both patient and professional.

A rating is allocated by overall dental attractiveness rather than specific morphological similarity to the photographs. The value arrived at gives an indication of the patient's treatment need on the grounds of aesthetic impairment, and by inference reflects the psychosocial need for orthodontic treatment.

According to Lunn et al.,[99] basic data of potential treatment need and demand is required when considering the use of the IOTN index as a public health tool and not details of the type of treatment. In this respect, scores of 4 and 5 in the dental health component clearly indicate a need for orthodontic treatment independent of the aesthetic judgement by the patient. Conversely, scores of 1 and 2 do not constitute treatment need. The difficulty arises for those children with a dental health component score of 3. In this situation, the use of the aesthetic component comes into play, more especially for children with a low awareness of their own dental appearance. The authors reported that the IOTN was easy to calibrate experienced dental epidemiologists.[99] The epidemiologists found it a quick, easy and enjoyable index to use (more so than DMF) and the index was readily accepted by children. There was a high level of agreement between examiners on the dental health component. The agreement for the aesthetic component with 10 choices was lower, although 96 % fell into the moderate agreement category. The recalibration exercise showed that the examiners had remained stable after work in the field, which is an important element in the use of any proposed epidemiological index.

In a comparative study Tang and So[100] used the Occlusal Index (OI)[78] and the Index of Orthodontic Treatment Need (IOTN)[7] to assess orthodontic treatment needs in a local population of Hong Kong. They concluded that both indices were highly reproducible but significant differences in the treatment need as assessed by these two indices did occur. For instance, the OI method suggested 60% of the subjects had either "good occlusions" or "no treatment need", whilst only 2% of the subjects were shown by the IOTN to have no need for treatment. This difference may have resulted through differences in weighting missing teeth. The IOTN puts a heavy weight on missing teeth in any quadrant. For example, when more than one tooth is missing in any quadrant, the treatment need is "very great". When the absence of one tooth in any quadrant results in tilting of adjacent teeth, the treatment need is also "great". The heavy weighting for missing teeth in posterior quadrants is questionable

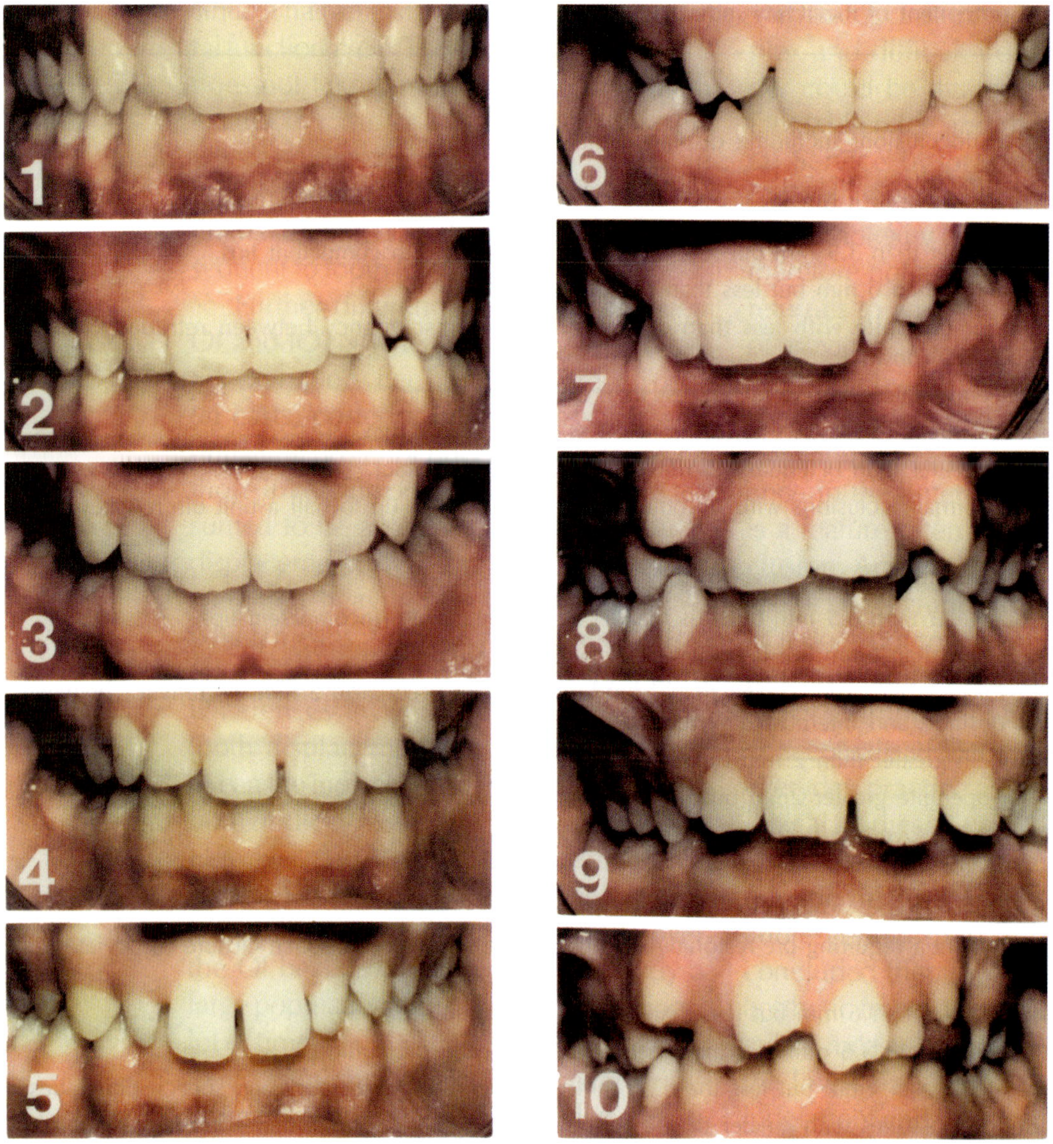

Fig. 4.1. The Dental Health Component of the IOTN index.
This component is reproduced by kind permission of The Victoria University of Manchester, England. These figures were first published in 1987 by European Orthodontic Society (Ruth Evans and William Shaw, Preliminary evaluation of an illustrated scale for rating dental attractiveness, European Journal of Orthodontics 9: 314-318).

treatment need on dental health grounds because of their greater knowledge of occlusion and experience with likely outcome.

The results of the Otuyemi et al.[103] study showed that some Nigerian adolescents encountered difficulty in matching their overall dental appearance, with specific reference to the morphological similarity on the aesthetic scale. For instance, a child with anterior openbite found it difficult to match their overall dental appearance, as this trait is not presented on the aesthetic scale. Phillips et al.[106] had earlier warned about the use of clinical photographs in determining the perception of dental attractiveness. The aesthetic component of the IOTN index may be criticised for its two-dimensional nature and its insufficiently wide range of dental appearances. Despite their criticism, Phillips et al.[106] reported a high correlation between the aesthetic and dental health components of the IOTN index.

Table 4.7. Components and weights of the Dental Aesthetic Index.

Component	Weight
Constant	13
Missing incisor, canine and premolar teeth – (number)	6
Crowding in incisal segments – number of segments crowded	1
Spacing in incisal segments number of segments crowded	1
Diastema – (mm)	3
Largest anterior irregularity, maxilla – (mm)	1
Largest anterior irregularity, mandible – (mm)	1
Anterior maxillary overjet – (mm)	2
Anterior mandible overjet – (mm)	4
Vertical anterior openbite – (mm)	4
Antero-posterior molar relation – largest deviation from normal either left or right, 0 = normal, 1 = 1/2 cusp either mesial or distal, 2 = 1 full cusp or more either mesial or distal	3
Total	**DAI score**

The aesthetic component of the IOTN index may not be sensitive enough to provide valid information on the psychosocial effects related to dental aesthetics. Firstly, there are only a few types of malocclusion represented in this scale of 10 photographs and usually people present with a larger range of occlusal conditions. Thus, it would be difficult to comprehensively rank the aesthetics of people with a wide range of different occlusal conditions from the information obtained from such a scale. The second limitation of this method is that it does not allow a view of the anteroposterior plane of the malocclusion (e.g., overjet), which is important for the assessment. Finally, it does not take into account issues such as the colour and shape of the teeth and missing teeth.

In Norway, a new orthodontic treatment need index was introduced by the National Health Insurance System.[107] As national subsidies for orthodontic care are limited, the government reimburses the treatment costs according to the severity of malocclusion. The Need for Orthodontic Treatment Index (NOTI)[107] defines four groups or grades, denoting "very great need", "great need", "obvious need", and "little/no need". Occlusal traits presumed to be associated with concern for dental appearance and psychosocial problems were incorporated in the index, but this was based solely on professional estimates. Selection of traits and definitions of cut-off points are based on present scientific evidence and empirical orthodontic norms about the risks for detrimental effects of dentofacial anomalies on dental health, function and psychosocial well-being.

Another recent development in assessing orthodontic treatment need is the Dental Aesthetic Index (DAI), which is an orthodontic index grounded in socially defined aesthetic norms.[84] It responds to the call for the inclusion of psychosocial factors in the assessment of malocclusion. The DAI allows the estimation of potential social handicaps if occlusal status deviates significantly from society's aesthetic norms. In contrast to other attempts to include aesthetic factors in assessment of malocclusion where separate assessments are made for the aesthetic and clinical components, the DAI links the aesthetic and clinical aspects of malocclusion into a single score.

The DAI recognises that socially derived norms for acceptable dental appearance sets the standard for evaluation of acceptable levels of dental aesthetics. It also recognises that the condition of malocclusion is socially defined by the deviation of occlusal configurations from social norms. Extreme deviations from acceptable dental appearance should have a negative impact on social, psychological and physical function. The DAI is an orthodontic index in the form of a regression equation that links the public's rating of the social acceptability of occlusal conditions with their clinically measured orthodontic traits. It was developed through the use of specially prepared photographs of 200 occlusal patterns that represented the wide range of untreated occlusal conditions found in a population of half a million adolescents.[84,108] The stimuli were completely neutral with regard to sex, race or ethnic origin. There were no confounding facial features that could influence subjects' assessment of facial acceptability of the stimuli. Stimuli were rated for social acceptability using a semantic differential instrument. Sixteen hundred students and adults in the USA participated in rating these stimuli. The resulting regression equation consisted of ten components of intraoral measurements of the morphological traits associated with dental aesthetics and their appropriate regression coefficients (weights). This regression equation is called the Standard DAI.

Table 7 represents the components of the Standard DAI regression equation, the actual and rounded regression coefficients (weights) for each component and the constant. The Standard DAI loses relatively little precision when regression weights are rounded. The higher the score on the DAI scale the more likely the untreated malocclusion will contribute to psychological, social or physical dysfunction. Depending on the DAI score an individual's occlusal status can then be classified into the following categories: normal occlusion or minor malocclusion, definite malocclusion with treatment elective, severe malocclusion with treatment highly desirable or handicapping malocclusion (Table 4.7).

The Peer Assessment Rating (PAR) Index developed by Richmond[109] and Richmond et al.[88] to measure treatment outcome takes into consideration occlusal changes, and has been found to be as reliable and valid as most other occlusal indices.[88,110] The PAR index is based on models of subjects and has no patient assessment of outcome. There are basically two methods of assessing improvement using the PAR Index: (1) reduction in the weighted PAR score and (2) percentage reduction in the weighted PAR score. This approach to evaluate orthodontic treatment outcome parallels the view of Berg (1991), who compared quantification of occlusion to general orthopaedics in medicine, where the degree of restitution of a handicap is frequently expressed as a percentage of the ideal. The PAR Index does not measure iatrogenic effects such as enamel lesions, marginal bone loss and apical root resorption as discussed by Linge and Linge.[111]

The concept of PAR is to assign a score

Table 4.8 Components of the PAR Index.

	Component
1	Upper right segment
2	Upper anterior segment
3	Upper left segment
4	Lower right segment
5	Lower anterior segment
6	Lower left segment
7	Right buccal occlusion
8	Overjet
9	Overbite
10	Centreline
11	Left buccal occlusion

to various occlusal traits that make up a malocclusion. The individual scores are summed to obtain an overall total, representing the degree to which a case deviates from normal alignment and occlusion. The score of zero indicates good alignment and higher scores (rarely beyond 50) indicate increased levels of irregularity. There are 11 components of the PAR Index (Table 4.8).

A new orthodontic index, the Index of Complexity Outcome and Need (ICON index), was developed by Daniels and Richmond[85] to assess treatment need, complexity, and outcome. The ICON index was designed for an ease and rapid application both clinically and on study models. It was validated using an international panel of orthodontists, who were asked to express their subjective opinion on the need for treatment, treatment complexity, the degree of occlusal improvement and the acceptability of a number of untreated and treated cases. It is valid in as much as it broadly represents the prevailing expert approach to treatment entry and exit thresholds. The ICON index contains 5 components: dental aesthetics, crossbite, anterior vertical relationship, upper arch crowding/spacing and buccal segment sagital relationship.

From the review so far it is reasonable to conclude that the development of an index to assess 'handicapping' malocclusion will not be possible until more objective methods of measuring the effect of a malocclusion on the individual's psychological and social need, are included. Furthermore, any evaluation of the effectiveness of health services should reveal to what extent the goals of providing care have been reached. Moreover, when evaluating orthodontic services one has to decide whose viewpoints are primarily considered, because the patient, provider, and purchaser may have different expectations concerning orthodontic treatment.[112] In addition, when orthodontic resources are limited, any evaluation must take into account the resources available to the service.

Oral impacts of malocclusion

The shift in emphasis from the clinical measures to the behavioural domain of oral health and to the development of sociodental indicators highlights a broader scope for oral health. The functional, social, psychological, cultural and economic effects of oral conditions, and not only the presence or absence of oral pathology, should be considered.[113] The shift in emphasis should be reflected in assessment of outcomes of orthodontic treatment.

In an early critical review of the impacts of oral conditions, Sheiham and Croog[114] acknowledged the importance of the oral region for physical health and social, psychological and economic well-being of individuals. They called for the comprehensive assessment of the impact of oral impacts on individuals and its complex implications for society. Clearly, the impacts of oral conditions and diseases cover wide domains of life, such as functional limitation, disability, interpersonal relations, social interaction, economic situation, work, family life and leisure activities, thus highlighting the influence of oral health on quality of life.[115,116]

Much research has been directed towards the assessment of impacts from malocclusion and more severe dentofacial anomalies. These conditions are not usually associated with limitation in the physical ability of the individual, unless there is a functional problem. Nevertheless, the social and psychological impacts are considerable. In the early 1970s, the need to explore these dimensions in defining and describing malocclusion became apparent.[117] At the same time, McGregor[118] raised the issue of stereotyping and potential handicap of dentofacial deformities in relation to self-image and social interaction, while Stricker,[119] in evaluating the psychological aspects of malocclusion, showed that the level of satisfaction with appearance was related to the self-esteem of the individual.

Current research indicates that unacceptable subjective dental appearance, including visible dental characteristics that deviate greatly from the norm, may stigmatise, impede career advancement and peer group acceptance, encourage negative stereotyping and have a negative effect on self-concept.[81] Dental appearance that deviates from acceptable norms might indeed reduce opportunities. For prestigious occupations, where dental appearance is important, and in which the person is visible to the public, an individual's dentofacial disorders may come between career aspirations and career opportunities.[84] Rosenberg[120] argued that social standards of appearance determine self-concept by affecting how people perceive themselves.

In a classic early study, individuals with cleft lip or palate were compared to their healthy siblings in relation to family life. Subjects with cleft lip or palate were less likely to marry. Furthermore, when they married, they did so at a later age, and were less likely to have children.[121] Apart from that, teachers rated less accurately the intellectual ability of children with facial deformities, in comparison to those without,[122] while there was evidence that lower academic expectations and more negative opinion about the behaviour and personality are attributes associated with children considered to be unattractive.[123]

Conversely, in a review of the literature on the social effects of malocclusion, Shaw et al.[2] failed to identify conclusive evidence regarding the assessment of dentofacial anomalies on daily life. However, they acknowledged the fact that unattractive physical appearance may be related to unfavourable social interaction. Although they suspected important handicapping effects in extreme cases of malocclusion, they concluded, "there is no specific, direct evidence that unfavourable stereotyping operates against individuals with visible dental irregularities or that it interferes with personal development".[59] A longitudinal study of children aged 11-12 years old also failed to demonstrate strong associations between measures of dental status, attractiveness and psychosocial well-being.[124] However, the authors accepted that the results might have been influenced by the choice of measures of psychological impact. In addition, the results may have been influenced by a relatively small sample of school children with severe forms of malocclusion as opposed to those attending orthodontic treatment. They further explained the lack of evidence linking malocclusion with social and psychological impacts, by suggesting that physical attractiveness may be less crucial to young children. The effects of malocclusion on psychological well-being may however become more obvious in later adolescence.

In another study of children aged 9-13 years, which assessed the extent of teasing and harassment caused by deviant dental characteristics, poor appearance of teeth and mouth was related to significant social handicap.[59] Teeth represented the fourth most frequent feature that related to teasing, followed by height, weight and hair. Children teased about their teeth were twice more likely to suffer general harassment and over 60% of them admitted that they disliked or were upset by it. The prevalence of teasing, combined with dissatisfaction about appearance, was reported to be significantly higher among Danish adolescents with malocclusion traits, mainly extreme maxillary overjet, extreme deep bite and space anomalies, in comparison to those who were not diagnosed for malocclusion.[97] In a methodologically challenging 15-year follow-up study of 30-year-olds Danes, that focused on specific conditions related to malocclusion both retrospectively and presently, the results showed that conspicuous occlusal anomalies and maxillary crowding adversely affected body image and self-concept in both adolescence and adulthood.[97]

A more detailed longitudinal study used various measurements in a two-year follow-up with the aim to evaluate the psychological changes related to orthognathic surgery in 46 patients, aged between 12 and 47 years.[125] They found that although oral function, pain and paresthesia decreased over time, self-esteem of patients fluctuated considerably. Self-esteem was higher before the operation, possibly due to an anticipation of desirable outcomes, but significantly lower nine months after the operation. Self-esteem increased again by the two-year follow-up but failed to reach pre-operative values. Nevertheless, overall and profile body images improved significantly and all patients reported high levels of satisfaction with the surgery. Satisfaction was related to their perception of aesthetic improvements, irrespective of the presence of functional problems.

The finding that some occlusal traits can create psychosocial problems suggests the desirability of incorporating psychosocial aspects into the professional reappraisal of criteria for treatment particularly when new indices are being developed. Even though indices are necessary instruments from an administrative point of view, they fail to indicate whether the malocclusion traits presented will have an adverse effect on the individual child. To resolve this dilemma, Helm[62] stated, "that profound psychological insight is required" as decisions "must be based on impressions of the child's personality and its personal resources in coping with a deviating dentofacial appearance".

It seems reasonable to postulate that the concept of "handicapping" malocclusions, although yet undefined, in some way involves the interrelations of the psychological effects on the child and the aesthetic impact of his appearance on his/her peers. If so, there may be no numerical index based on occlusal morphology alone that will be an effective substitute for the personal evaluation of each applicant by the clinician.[62] Indeed, there is now general agreement within the orthodontic profession that a clinical determination of "need for treatment" should include consideration of the psychosocial, as well as the physical, effects of malocclusion.[62] However, neither psychosocial effects of malocclusion nor psychosocial responses to orthodontic treatment have been demonstrated in systematic research. Moreover, in recent years, the use of public funds to provide orthodontic treatment has emphasised the need to verify the deleterious psychological and social effects of malocclusion and determine the degree to which they are alleviated by orthodontic treatment.

Oral conditions affect many areas of life, including work, family life, economics and social interactions, but the larger implications of these social and psychological effects on society have rarely been examined.[114] The impact of oral health problems on society is usually measured by outcomes related to limitations in role performance and functional capabilities. Such broadly based indicators are multidimensional measures that assess the social, psychological and economic impacts of oral disorders on society.[113]

Conclusions

Thus, need for orthodontic treatment may only be assessed in absolute terms with accurate information regarding the long-term effects of malocclusion. Currently, this information is unavailable. However, in the absence of clear evidence, it would seem reasonable to introduce a structured index, i.e., IOTN, to enable a uniform approach to assess treatment need which can be modified in the light of new evidence. There are many other factors that are considered when assessing orthodontic treatment need. However, the importance of these factors has yet to be quantified and prioritised.

Until an approach to objectively assess orthodontic treatment need is accepted and used by the profession, the distortion of the need and demand for orthodontic treatment by dentists' unequal perceptions will continue.

Orthodontic services are an interesting aspect of dental public health. Malocclusion is not a disease but rather a set of dental variations that have, in the main, a limited influence upon oral health. Yet demand for services in most countries generally exceeds supply and presents difficult choices in the distribution of public health resources. The use of indices to target resources and secure an adequate risk-cost balance is desirable. Furthermore, within the context of a public dental health system, where it is preferable that allocation of resources is based on need rather than demand, the use of the IOTN index will assist those responsible for planning, contracting and monitoring orthodontic services in the UK.

References

1. Foster TD, Menezes DM. The assessment of occlusal features for public health planning purposes. *Am J Orthod Dentofacial Orthop*, 1976;69:83-90.
2. Shaw WC, Gabe MJ, Jones BM. The expectations of orthodontic patients in South Wales and St. Louis, Missouri. *Br J Orthod*, 1980;7:75-80.
3. Foster TD. Orthodontic surveys – a critical appraisal. *Br J Orthod*, 1980; 7:59-63.
4. Shaw WC, O'Brien KD, Richmond S, Brook P. Quality control in Orthodontics: risk/benefit considerations. *Br Dent J*, 1991; 170(1):33-37.
5. Shaw WC, O'Brien KD, Richmond S. Quality control in orthodontics: Factors influencing the receipt of orthodontic treatment. *Br Dent J*, 1991;170:66-68.
6. Shaw WC, O'Brien KD, Richmond S, Brook P. Quality control in orthodontics: Indices of treatment need and treatment demands. *Br Dent J*, 1991;170:107-111.
7. Brook PH, Shaw WC. The development of an orthodontic priority index. *Eur J Orthod*, 1989;11:309-320.
8. Draker HL. Handicapping labio-lingual conditions: a proposed index for public health purposes. *Am J Orthod Dentofacial Orthop*, 1960;46:295-305.
9. Tulloch J FC, Shaw WC, Smith A. A comparison of attitudes toward orthodontic treatment in British and American communities. *Am J Orthod Dentofacial Orthop* 1984;85:253-259.
10. Stephens CD, Orton HS, Usiskin LA. Future manpower requirements for orthodontics undertaken in the general dental services. *Br J Orthod*, 1985;12:168-175.
11. Chiavaro A. Malocclusion of the temporary teeth. *Int J Orthod*,1915;1:171-179.
12. Korkhans G. The frequency of orthodontic anomalies at various ages. *Int J Orthod*, 1928;14:120-135.
13. Hill IN, Balayney JR, Wolf W. Prevalence of malocclusion of children in a fluoridated and control area. *J Dent Res*, 1959;38:782-794.
14. Gardiner JH. An orthodontic survey of Libyan schoolchildren. *Br J Orthod* 1982;1:59-61.
15. Hirschwitz AS, Rahid S, Cleaton PE. Dental caries, gingival health and malocclusion in 12 years old urban black schoolchildren from Soweto, Johannesburg. *Community Dent Oral Epidemiol*, 1981;9:87-90.
16. Sclare R. Orthodontics and the school child: a survey of 680 children. *Br Dent J*, 1945;79:278-280.
17. Bjork A. The face in profile. *Swed Dent J*, 1974;40 Suppl 5B.
18. Massler M, Frankel JM. Prevalence of malocclusion in children aged 14 to 18 years. *Am J Orthod Dentofacial Orthop*, 1951;37:751-768.
19. Telle ES. A study of the frequency of malocclusion in the country of Hedmark, Norway. *Trans Eur Orthod*, Soc 1951; 25:192-198.
20. Gardiner JH. A survey of malocclusion and some aetiological factors in 1000 Sheffield schoolchildren. *Dent Pract Dent Rec*, 1956;6:187-198.
21. Goose DH, Thomson A, Winter F. Ma-

locclusion in schoolchildren of the West Midland. *Br Dent J*, 1957;102:174-178.
22. Altemus LA. The frequency of the incidence of malocclusion in American children aged 12-18 years. *Angle Orthod*, 1959;29:189-200.
23. Breham H, Jackson D. An investigation of the extent of the need for orthodontic services. *Am J Orthod Dentofacial Orthop*, 1961;47:148-149.
24. Haynes S. The prevalence of malocclusion in English schoolchildren aged 11-12 years. *Trans Eur Orthod Soc*, 1970; 48:89 98.
25. Foster TD, Walpole AJ. A survey of malocclusion and the need for orthodontic treatment in Shropshire schoolchildren. *Br J Orthod*, 1974;1:73-78.
26. Robert EE, Goose DH. Malocclusion in a North Wales population. *Br Dent J*, 1979;146:17-20.
27. Isiekwe MC. Malocclusion in Lagos, Nigeria. *Community Dent Oral Epidemiol*, 1982;11:59-62.
28. Abbu-Affan A, Wisth P, Boe O. Malocclusion in 12 year old Sudanese children. *Trop Dent J*, 1990;13:87-93.
29. Richardson A, Ana JR. Occlusion and malocclusion in Lagos. *J Dent*, 1973;1: 134-139.
30. Muniz BR. Epidemiology of malocclusion in Argentine children. *Community Dent Oral Epidemiol*, 1986;14:221-224.
31. Silva Filho OG, Freitas SF, Cavassan AO. Prevalence of normal occlusion and malocclusion in Bauru (Sao Paulo) students. Influence of socio-economic level. *Rev Odontol Univ São Paulo*, 1990;4 (3):189-196.
32. El-Mangoury NH, Mostafa YA. Epidemiological panorama of dental occlusion. *Angle Orthod*, 1990;60(3): 207-214.
33. Baume LJ. Uniform methods for the epidemiological assessment of malocclusion. Results obtained with the World Health Organisation standard methods (1962 and 1971) in South Pacific populations. *Am J Orthod Dentofacial Orthop*, 1974;66:251-272.
34. Helm S. Malocclusion in Danish children with adolescent dentition: an epidemiological study. *Am J Orthod Dentofacial Orthop*, 1968;54:352-368.
35. Lundstrom A, Lundstrom O. A dental examination of the mixed and permanent dentition in a Nubian population. *Acta Odontol Scand*, 1969;27: 371-386.
36. Nashashibi I, Darwish SK, Kalifa EL. Prevalence of malocclusion and treatment needs in Riyadi (Saudi Arabia). *Odonto-Stomatologie Tropicale*, 1983; 6:209-214.
37. Steigman S, Kawar M, Zilberman Y. Prevalence and severity of malocclusion in Israel Arab-urban children 13 to 15 years of age. *Am J Orthod Dentofacial Orthop*, 1983;84:337-343.
38. Farawana NW. Malocclusion in Iraq. *Quintessence Int*, 1987;18(2):153-157.
39. Jacobson A. Occlusion and malocclusion in the South African Bantu. *J Dent South Africa*, 1967;22:300-307.
40. Kapila S. Distribution of malocclusion in African and Asian children in Nairobi schools. *Odonto-Stomatologie Tropicale*, 1983;6:209-214.
41. Garner LD, Butt MH. Malocclusion in black Americans and Nyeri Kenyans. An epidemiological study. *Angle Orthod*, 1985;2:139-146.
42. Diagne F, Ba I, Ba-Diop K, Yam AA, Ba-Tamba A. Prevalence of malocclusion in Senegal. *Community Dent Oral Epidemiol*, 1993;22:325-326.
43. Kerosuo H, LaineT, Kerosuo E, Ngassapa D, Honkala E. Occlusion among a group of Tanzanian urban schoolchildren. *Community Dent Oral Epidemiol*, 1988; 16:306-309.
44. Grewe JM, Cervenka J, Shapiro BL, Witkop CJ. Prevalence of malocclusion in Chippewa Indian children. *J Dent Res*, 1968;47:302-305.
45. Horowitz HS. A study of occlusal relations in 10- to 12-year-old Caucasian and Negro children. Int Dent J 1970;20:593-605.
46. Ingervall B. Prevalence and occlusal anomalies in Swedish conscripts. *Acta Odontol Scand*, 1974;32:83-92.
47. Laine T, Hausen H. Occlusal anomalies in Finnish students related to age, sex, absent permanent teeth and orthodontic treatment. *Eur J Orthod*, 1983;5:125-131.
48. Salzmann JA. Malocclusion and treatment need in the United States youths 12-17 years of age. *Am J Orthod Dentofacial Orthop*, 1977;72:579-581.
49. Siriwat PP, Jarabak JR. Malocclusion and facial morphology. Is there a relationship? - An epidemiologic study. *Angle Orthod*, 1985;55:127-138.
50. Solow B, Helm S. A method for tabulation and statistical evaluation of epidemio-

logic malocclusion data. *Acta Odontol Scand,* 1968;26:63-88.
51. Wood BF. Malocclusion in the modern Alaskan Eskimo. *Am J Orthod Dentofacial Orthop,* 1971;60:344-354.
52. Angle EH. Classification of malocclusion. *Dental Cosmos,* 1899;41:248-264.
53. Shaw WC, Addy J, Ray C. Dental and social effects of malocclusion and effectiveness of orthodontic treatment: A review. *Community Dent Oral Epidemiol,* 1980;8:36-45.
54. Graber TM. *Orthodontics: principles and practice.* 3rd ed. Philadelphia: WB Saunders Co.; 1972.
55. Sadowsky C, BeGole EA. Long-term status of temporomandibular joint function and functional occlusion after orthodontic treatment. *Am J Orthod Dentofacial Orthop,* 1980;78:201-12.
56. Sadowsky C, BeGole, E.A. Long-term effects of orthodontic treatment on periodontal health. *Am J Orthod Dentofacial Orthop,* 1981;80:156-172.
57. Ramfjord SP, Ash MM. Significance of occlusion in the etiology and treatment of early, moderate and advanced periodontitis. *J Periodontol,* 1981; 52:511-517.
58. Bell R, Kiyak HA, Joondeph DR, McNeil RW, Wallen TR. Perceptions of facial profile and their influence on the decision to undergo orthognathic surgery. *Am J Orthod Dentofacial Orthop,* 1985; 88:323-332.
59. Shaw WC. The social implications of dentofacial deformities. PhD Thesis. University of Wales; 1980.
60. Isaacson RJ. In response - oral health in the United States: prevalence of malocclusion. *J Dent Educ,* 1985; 49:397.
61. Prahl-Andersen B. The need for orthodontic treatment. *Angle Orthod,* 1978;48:1-9.
62. Helm S. Reappraisal of the criteria for orthodontic treatment. PhD Thesis. Oslo: University of Oslo; 1990.
63. Proffit WR. Contemporary orthodontics. St Louis (MO): C.V. Mosby; 1986.
64. Solow B. Guest editorial: orthodontic screening and third party financing. *Eur J Orthod,* 1995;17:79-83.
65. World Health Organization. *Oral Health Care Systems: An international collaborative study.* London. Quintessence; 1985.
66. Downer MC. Craniofacial anomalies – are they a public health problem? *Int Dent J,* 1987;37:193-196.
67. Salzmann JA. Handicapping malocclusion assessment to establish treatment priority. *Am J Orthod Dentofacial Orthop,* 1968; 54:749-765.
68. British Dental Association (UK). Memorandum on Orthodontic Services. London: BDA; 1954.
69. Relman AS. Assessment and accountability: The third revolution in health care. *New England J Med,* 1988; 319(18):1220.
70. Vig KWL, Bennett ME, O'Brien K, Vayda D, Vig PS, Weyant RJ. Orthodontic process and outcome: efficacy and effectiveness studies. *In:* McNamara JA Jr, Trotman C, Ferrara A (ed). *Orthodontic Treatment: Outcome and Effectiveness,* Vol. 30. Craniofacial Growth Series, Center for Human Growth and Development, The University of Michigan, Ann Arbor, Michigan; 1994.
71. Stallard H. The general prevalence of gross symptoms of malocclusion. *Dental Cosmos,* 1932;74:29-37.
72. McCall JD. A study of malocclusion in preschool and school children. *Dental Items of Interest,* 1944;131-133.
73. Van Kirk LK, Pennel EH. Assessment of malocclusion in population groups. *Am J Orthod Dentofacial Orthop,* 1959;45 (10):752-758.
74. Fisk RO. When malocclusion concerns the public. *Can Dent Assoc,* 1960;26(7):397- 412.
75. Grainger RM. *Malocclusion severity estimate.* Burlington Orthodontic Research Centre. Progress Report; 1960. Series V1: 9-11.
76. Poulton DR, Aaronson SA. The relationship between occlusion and periodontal status. *Am J Orthod Dentofacial Orthop* 1961;47(9):690-699.
77. Bjork A, Krebs A, Solow B. A method for epidemiological registration of malocclusion. *Acta Odontol Scand,* 1964; 22(1): 27-41.
78. Summers CJ. The Occlusal Index: a system for identifying and scoring occlusal disorders. *Am J Orthod Dentofacial Orthop,* 1971;59:552-567.
79. Grainger RM. Orthodontic Treatment Priority Index. Public Health Service, Washington DC: United Stated Government, Printing office; 1967. Publication number 1000, series 2, number 25.
80. Profitt WR, Ackerman JL. Rating the characteristics of malocclusion: a syste-

matic approach for planning treatment. *Am J Orthod Dentofacial Orthop,* 1973;64(3): 258-269.

81. Linder Aronson S. Orthodontics in the Swedish public health system. *Trans Eur Orthod Soc,* 1974;233-240.
82. Brzroukov V, Freer TJ, Helm S, Kalamkarov H, Sardoinfirri J, Solow B. Basic methods for recording malocclusion traits. *Bull of World Health Organisation,* 1979;57 (6):955-961.
83. Kinaar BK, Burker PH. Quantitative assessment of the occlusal features. *Br J Orthod,* 1981;8:149-156.
84. Cons NC, Jenny J, Kohout FJ. *DAI: the Dental Aesthetic Index.* Iowa City, Iowa: College of Dentistry, University of Iowa; 1986.
85. Daniels C, Richmond S. The development of the Index of Complexity, Outcome and Need (ICON). *J Orthod,* 2000; 27(2):149-162.
86. Richmond S, Shaw WC, O'Brien K, Buchanan IB, Stephens CD, Andrews M, Roberts CT. The relationship between IOTN and the consensus opinion of a panel of 74 dentists. *Br Dent J,* 1995; 178:370-374.
87. Stenvik A. Orthodontic care: need and demand. PhD Thesis. Oslo, University of Oslo; 1997.
88. Richmond S, Shaw WC, Stephens CD, O'Brien KD, Buchanan IB, Jones R, Roberts CT, Andrews, M. The development of the Par Index (Peer Assessment Rating), reliability and validity. *Eur J Orthod,* 1992;14:125-139.
89. Salzmann JA. Treatment priority index of malocclusion. *Int Dent J,* 1970;20:618-630.
90. Carlos JP. Evaluation of indices of malocclusion. *Int Dent J,* 1970;20:606-617.
91. Helm S. Intra-examiner reliability of epidemiological registrations of malocclusion. *Acta Odontol Scand,* 1977; 35:161-165.
92. Barmes DE. The orthodontic problem: a global perspective. *Trans Eur Orthod Soc,* 1973;465-70.
93. World Health Organization. *Standardization of reporting of dental diseases and conditions, report of an expert committee on dental health.* Geneva: World Health Organization; 1962. Technical Report Series, 242.
94. World Health Organization. *Oral Health Surveys: Basic Methods.* Geneva: World Health Organization; 1971.
95. Sheiham A, Spencer J. Health needs assessment. *In:* Pine CM (ed). *Community Oral Health.* Oxford: Reed Educational & Professional Publishing Ltd; 1997. p. 39-54.
96. Shaw WC. The influence of children's dentofacial appearance on their social attractiveness judged by peers and lay adults. *Am J Orthod Dentofacial Orthop,* 1981;79:399-415.
97. Helm S, Kreibord S, Solow B. Psychosocial implications of malocclusion: a 15-year follow-up study in 30-year-old Danes. *Am J Orthod Dentofacial Orthop,* 1985;87:110-118.
98. Espeland LV, Gronlund G, Stenvik A. Concern for dental appearance among Norwegian young adults in region with low uptake of orthodontic treatment. *Community Dent Oral Epidemiol,* 1993; 21.
99. Lunn H, Richmond S, Mitropoulos C. The use of the Index of Orthodontic Treatment Need (IOTN) as a public Health tool: a pilot study. *Community Dent Health,* 1993;10:111-121.
100. Tang ELK, So LLY. A comparative study using the Occlusal Index and the Index of Orthodontic Treatment Need. *Angle Orthod,* 1993;63(1):57-64.
101. Elias AC, Sheiham A. The relationship between satisfaction with mouth and number and position of teeth - Review. *J Oral Rehabil,* 1998;25:649-661.
102. de Oliveira CM. The use of the Index of Orthodontic Treatment Need (IOTN) for planning, contracting and monitoring orthodontic services. MSc Thesis. Department of Epidemiology and Public Health, University College London, University of London; 1997.
103. Otuyemi OD, Veboko VI, Adekoya-Sofowora CA, Ndukwe KC. Unmet orthodontic treatment need in rural Nigerian adolescents. *Community Dent Oral Epidemiol,* 1997;25:363-366.
104. Shaw WC, Luis HG, Robertson NRE. Perception of malocclusion. *Br Dent J,* 1975;138:211-216.
105. Holmes A. The subjective need and demand for orthodontic treatment need. *Br J Orthod,* 1992;19:287-297.
106. Phillips C, Tulloch C, Donn C. Rating of

facial attractiveness. *Community Dent Oral Epidemiol,* 1992;20:214-20.

107. Espeland LV, Ivarsson K, Stenvik A. A new Norwegian index of orthodontic treatment need related to orthodontic concern among 11-year-olds and their parents. *Community Dent Oral Epidemiol,* 1992;20:274-279.
108. Ast DB, Carlos JP, Cons NC. The prevalence and characteristics of malocclusion among senior high school students in upstate New York. *Am J Orthod Dentofacial Orthop,* 1965; 51:437-45.
109. Richmond S. A critical evaluation of orthodontic treatment in the General Dental Services of England and Wales. PhD thesis. University of Manchester (UK); 1990.
110. Buchanan IB, Shaw WC, Richmond S, O'Brien KD, Andrews M. A comparison of the reliability and validity of the PAR Index and Summer' Occlusal Index. *Eur J Orthod,* 1993;15:27-31.
111. Linge L, Linge BO. Patient characteristics and treatment variables associated with root resorption during orthodontic treatment. *Am J Orthod Dentofacial Orthop,* 1991;99:35-43.
112. Howatt A. Orthodontics and health: have we widened our perspectives? *Community Dent Health,* 1993;10:Supplement 2,29-37.
113. Reisine ST, Locker D. Social, psychological and economic impacts of dental conditions and treatments. In: Cohen LK, Gift HC (ed). *Disease Prevention and Oral Health Promotion: Sociodental Sciences in Action.* Copenhagen: Munksgaard; 1995. p. 33-71.
114. Sheiham A, Croog SH. The psychological impact of dental diseases on individuals and communities. *J Behav Med,* 1981; 4:257-271.
115. Nikias MK. Oral disease and the quality of life. *Am J Public Health,* 1985;75:11-12.
116. Miller WA. Does oral health influence quality of life? *Gerodontics,* 1987;3:99.
117. Cohen L, Horowitz HS. Occlusal relations in children born and reared in an opitmally fluoridated community, III. Social-psychological findings. *Angle Orthod,* 1970;40:159-169.
118. McGregor F. Social and psychological implications of dentofacial disfigurement. *Angle Orthod,* 1970;40:231-233.
119. Stricker G. Psychological issues pertaining to malocclusion. *Am J Orthod Dentofacial Orthop,* 1970;58:276-283.
120. Rosenberg M. *Malocclusion and craniofacial malformation: self-concept implications. Paper presented at the workshop on psychosocial aspects of craniofacial malformation.* Hilton Head, SC; 1974.
121. Peter JP, Chinsky RR. Sociological aspects of cleft palate adults, I: Marriage. *Cleft Palate Craniofac J,* 1974;11:295-309.
122. Richman LC. The effects of facial disfigurement on teacher's perception of ability in cleft palate children. *Cleft Palate Craniofac J,* 1978;15:155-160.
123. Baldwin DC. Appearance and aesthetics in oral health. *Community Dent Oral Epidemiol,* 1980;8:244-56.
124. Kenealy P, Frude N, Shaw WC. The influence of social class on the uptake of orthodontic treatment. *Br J Orthod,* 1989;16:107-111.
125. Kiyak HA, Hohl T, West RA, McNeill RW. Psychological changes in orthognathic surgery patients: a 24 month follow-up. *J Oral Maxillofac Surg,* 1984;42:506-512.

Chapter 5

Healthy Environments: Strategies for Promotion of Children´s Oral Health

Simone Tetu Moysés
Cecile Soriano Rodrigues

Introduction

Health promotion is an important component of public policies. Health promotion represents a realistic perspective for the improvement of health of the whole population. The fundamental basis is centered on the wide conception of the process from health to disease and the determinants. Once the determinants have been identified they are incorporated into strategic planning. Health promotion definitions[1,2] in general accept that the individual (lifestyle) and structural elements (physical/social environment) form the critical portion of any strategy of health promotion.[3] Essentially, lifestyle approaches focus on the identification and reduction of risk behaviours associated with morbidity and premature deaths. The approach involves legislative (e.g. obligation to have safe seatbelts in cars), fiscal (higher taxes for cigarettes and alcohol), and social (food, sanitation, housing, and income policies) measures. This chapter approaches the strategy of creating environments that are favourable to health and outlines the implications for the oral health promotion of children. Initially, conceptual and practical fields of this strategy will be briefly highlighted. Next, influences of social and environmental factors in particular will be reviewed as determinants for general and oral health. Key elements of evidence about the effects of environmental measures on health will be explained. Health promotion interventions within the school context and the oral health promotion in preschool settings will also be critically evaluated.

The establishment of healthy environments

The *establishment of healthy environments* has a very high priority for action in health promotion[2,4,5,6,7,8] (Box 5.1). The term "environment" incorporates not only the "physical or natural" dimension, but also cultural, social, political, and economic dimensions. Under this perspective, health is seen as "the magnitude by which an individual or a group can, on one hand, accomplish its aspirations, and, on the other, change its environment and confront it".[9]

Box 5.1 Fields of action in health promotion.

1. **Healthy public policies** – to stimulate all policy makers, within and outside of the health sector, with the explicit concern with health and equity in all fields of public policies with an impact on health, making the healthy choices the easier ones.
2. **Establishment of favourable environments to health** - to develop health promotion actions in social spaces, creating life and working conditions that lead to health and well being.
3. **Strengthening of community action** – health can only be warranted and sustained when the community acquires control over its health.
4. **Development of personal abilities** – health promotion stimulates the personal development by means of the access to health information and education, developing in the individuals or groups the necessary competencies and abilities so that they are apt to make healthy choices.
5. **Reorientation of health services** – to encourage health services to have as a basis new paradigms of health, aimed to the prevention and health promotion.

The establishment of healthy environments allows people to acquire more control over their own health by building of contexts, behaviours, and social relations favourable to health and human development. It is not feasible to markedly improve other health determinants such as human biology, lifestyle, and services organization, without changing the "environment", since all are inseparably linked to the conditions for living.[10] Actions towards the establishment of healthy environments are resources applicable to life in social spaces where people live, study or work. Strategies in oral health policies for children must incorporate this new perspective, adopting strategies that emphasize the establishment of healthy environments. Strategies that make healthy choices the easier ones and unhealthy choices more difficult.

Promoting health, therefore, demands that people and organizations assume their role in the establishment of social environments that support healthy opportunities and choices, making the political commitment to sustainable development and the reduction of social and health inequalities explicit.

In the context of health promotion for children, healthy environments refer to the physical and social aspects that surround them. They involve the places where they live, the local communities, their houses, where they study and play. They include also the structure that determines their access to resources for life maintenance and the warranty of the right to health and citizenship, by the mutual and responsible development of self-esteem and autonomy.[6]

Social and environmental factors as health determinants

Some people still believe that health of children is basically a matter of keeping them clean, and preventing them from becoming sick. However, their health involves dimensions much wider than hygiene or "absence of diseases". It also involves: physical health: it is necessary to feel well and healthy; mental and emotional health: it is necessary to be happy and balanced, able to use efficiently one's mind and body; social health, besides individual health: children need to live collectively, in cooperative environments where they are respected. They should have access to appropriate learning opportunities. In addition, everyone should have the warranty of equal rights and opportunities. Last, environmental health. If the environment is polluted, then clean food, water and air should be made available.[11]

Health promotion, therefore, highlights the fundamental need to recognize wider determinants of health. Theoretical models explaining health determinants that reinforce the interrelation and interdependence between social and cultural factors, on one hand, and environmental, structural, and material ones, on the other hand, have directly influenced those public health actions towards the child population in the past decades. The model proposed by Dahlgren and Whitehead[12] (Fig. 5.1) outlines how individual factors, including biological and life style aspects, are related to the social and community support offered by the family, care providers, friends and other significant elements within the local community. The individual factors are directly influenced by life and working conditions, including housing, income, and access to services, which are determined by wider social and economic conditions, such as economic development, public policies, social, cultural and environmental forces. Under this perspective, promoting health involves the development of actions that alter these determinants.

The contemporary discussion about inequalities and iniquities in health has also demonstrated the influence of social, economic, and environmental conditions on health, including oral health. Even though they are, in general, considered as synonyms, the expressions social inequality and inequity in health have their different meanings. While social inequality in health refers to any disparity observed on health conditions between groups, cities, and countries, social inequity gives prominence to the aspect of injustice in these differences.

"Promoting equity and decreasing iniquity requires not only a process of continuous equalization, but also a process of abolishment and decreasing of privileges."[13]

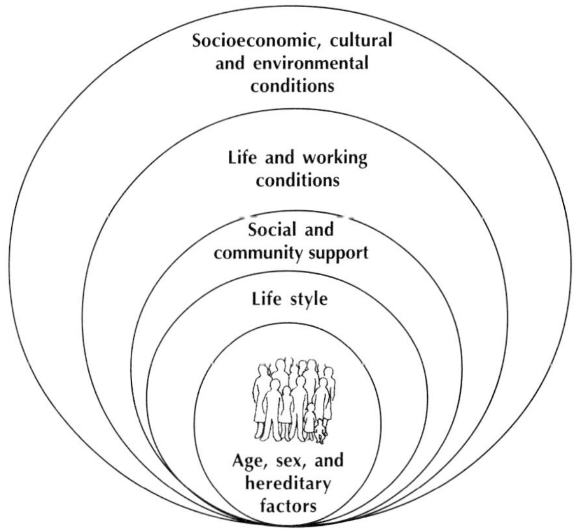

Fig. 5.1. Main determinants of health (Dahlgren and Whitehead, 1992).

The concept of social iniquity in health is particularly important for the understanding of epidemiological standards and stands to the social justice and to how much the recognition of fundamental human rights potentially promotes health (Box 5.2).

Box 5.2. Reference milestones for the understanding of equity and health.

- **Human Rights** – according to the Universal Declaration of Human Rights, published in 1948, "everyone is born free and equal in dignity and rights."

  In Brazil, the Child and Adolescent Statute (Brazil, 1990; Federal Law 8.669 / 1990) declares, in its Chapter 2, Art. 7º, that:

  "The child and the adolescent have right to life and health protection, by means of the effectiveness of public social policies that allows the healthy harmonic birth and development, in worthy conditions of existence."
- **Social Justice** – it explicitly analyzes who benefits – or is harmed – with the economic exploitation, iniquity and natural resources degradation.

In studies that relate socioeconomic conditions and health focusing on the dental caries experience, there is a consistently higher prevalence of caries in children of low socioeconomic condition.[14,15,16] In the United Kingdom, for example, even though oral health have improved, inequalities in oral health increased, mainly among preschool children. Forty percent of the children between 1 and 4 years of age from low socioeconomic conditions have experienced dental caries, while only 16% of the children from families with a better socioeconomic condition had caries.[17,18] Inequalities in oral health will only be reduced with an effective and appropriate policy of health promotion, which must have as a focus, the determinants of oral diseases. In Brazil, a country with big contrasts, [19] many studies have confirmed the effects of socioeconomic conditions on the prevalence of dental caries, dental trauma and pain in children and adolescents.[19,20,21,22]

Besides socioeconomic conditions, other aspects may define the patterns of health and disease of Brazilian children. Moysés[23] analyzed how intra-urban differences affected oral health in children. They related to indicators of public healthy policy implementation in some low income regions in Curitiba. Oral health depended on the micro areas where the children lived, characterized by different levels of implementation of public policies in fields like education, health, food, and housing.

There is unanimity in recommending the adoption of health promotion strategies involving public policies as a way to reduce inequalities. Promoting the health of children, therefore, implies expanding actions beyond the individual and standards of behaviour. This means recognizing that environmental conditions may differentially affect the health of children. The relationship between the child and the environment are characterized by cycles of interacting influences, in which physical and social characteristics of the community, the school and the family, and closer environments where they develop their daily experiences, directly influence their health at the same time as their own individual and collective actions in these environments modify their ability to achieve health.[24,25]

Social support as an element of children's health promotion

Social support refers to the comradeship and practical and informational support, as well as the esteem derived from the interaction of individuals with members of their social network, including friends, colleagues, acquaintances and family members.[26] The social support created in the environments where children live, such as their house, the day care centre, the school, the community, becomes essential for the building their health. Social support influences health and well being by two main mechanisms: first, by means of a direct effect on health; second, operating through the "buffering" effect, controlling stressor factors, like psychosocial adversities.[27,28,29,30,31,32]

Direct effects on health can be mediated by behaviours linked to health. The support provided by people from the family or important people at school or in the community may encourage children to assume healthy behaviours. Direct effects on health may also result from the social support through the widening of the perception of control over the environment, reinforcing self-confidence - that improves well being and immunity to diseases. On the other hand, the "buffering" effect may act when the support of another person may moderate the impact of the stressor agent, helping the person to control its consequences, and thereby enhance or maintain health.[31] In this way, actions for strengthening interpersonal relationships such as towards violence control inside the school, for example, may have an important impact on children's health.

The health of children and the family environment

Changes in family life and in social policies during the last decades have oriented public awareness about what families can and should now do for their members.[33] The family is considered a powerful social space to promote physical and emotional well being. It plays an important role in prevention and control of diseases, influencing concepts about health and disease of children, health behaviours, prevention and fighting diseases. Family influences affective, cognitive, and behavioural responses are directly related to general and oral health promotion. Fear, values, and the importance related to appropriate dental care, beliefs about oral health and how people establish and maintain self care, oral hygiene habits, and a healthy diet are some examples of practices forged within the family.[34]

The way families support or promote health among children is influenced by several principles and mechanisms related to family functions, abilities, and structural characteristics. Pratt[35] makes a distinction between the structure and family support functions. The structure is considered "organizational and properties and abilities that allow families to offer support to healthy health practices." These aspects include long lasting relationships, frequent and regular contacts among members, good relationships, accessibility among the members, normative prescriptions of shared responsibilities, and common location at home, where basic activities of health support and maintenance are accomplished. In this way, a house with two parents, instead of one only, household division of tasks, methods for raising children, and the employment condition of the mother are considered important characteristics related to health and to health behaviour of children.[35,36]

Family functions are "the dynamics or mechanisms by which families provide support for the health practices of its members."[35] This includes links that the family establishes with external groups and resources that can support activities and needs of its members; the provision of company for activities; the support of information offered by the family; the model copied from parents and the ability to inculcate social norms, values, and cultural symbols that influence practices of care for the body by the process of socialization. Therefore, family is an important source of social support to its members.

Family offers support when it creates the necessary environment for a healthy life, increasing self-esteem and confidence, creating opportunities of access to goods, equipments and time that facilitate health practices and providing necessary information for healthier choices. On the other hand, social context of the family, that determines the circumstances where family and environment interact, are crucial for the support forged in the family. Social networks can be particularly important in the context of material deprivation circumstances to give support to mechanisms of control over certain determinants of health and disease.[37]

So, the establishment of public policies centred on the support to the family nucleus will be an important strategy for the health promotion of children.

School as a social space for health promotion

Schools have goals to educate students by the development of academic or cognitive abilities and by the transmission of knowledge, besides individual and social abilities that help in the building of their lives and in the contribution to other's lives with whom they are related.[38] Being social institutions, schools must be environments of conviviality, where personal, creative, and autonomous interaction guides education, action, participation, and self help by means of critical and awareness and liberty.[39,40] As highlighted by Setúbla,[41] school is not the only place to build citizenship, but the development of individuals and societies depends on the quality and opportunities of equalitarian education.

The school space may be conducive to the development of a healthy lifestyle, contributing for the establishment and maintenance of health of its staff, students, and local communities. Schools' social and physical environment can be improved to give support to health, combining actions in classroom with changes of the school environment, as well as involving families and communities.[8,42-45] Jointly with families, schools are essential spaces for the individual and social development.

The idea of promoting health in schools is not new. Beattie[46] described how schools, since 1900, are used as spaces for testing of public health interventions. Medical counselling, as part of sanitary principles instituted by means of the inspection of children, physical exams, and the introduction of school meals, were strategies introduced during the first half of the XXth century to establish personal health and hygiene. From the 1950's to the 1990's, the focus of actions was on the lifestyle of students and on the psychosocial origins of risk behaviours, such as smoking, drug use and sexual relations.

From social control to the control of their own health, education in health was accomplished in schools in the whole world. For several years, programmes of health promotion were implemented in the form of traditional health education through the school curriculum. Teachers should present information about behavioural risks to health hoping to provide the necessary knowledge to influence children's behaviour. These practices were based on a prescriptive and coercive model of education, focusing the reproduction of values and behaviours instead of a participatory process, generator of opportunities for the personal and collective well being and growth, offering an opportunity to exert control over their own health.[47]

Even though during the 1980's some school programmes have incorporated innovative methods for the development of abilities and attitudes to support students to make healthy lifestyle choices, actions of health education had minimal and short term effects.[43,48] Evidence from systematic literature reviews about oral health education programmes using traditional methods reinforce this assertion.[49,50,51,52]

An important element to make the school an environment for the positive learning and for the construction of life seems to be the establishment of a space that explicitly supports physical, emotional, and social well being of it students, besides their academic performance. Therefore, the efforts of health promotion for children should not be exclusively linked to the development of programmes specific to health behaviours, like smoking, diet or tooth brushing, but they should also take into consideration the total school environment to which children are daily exposed. The "Healthy School" described by Young and Williams,[53] brings the scope beyond the limits of the formal curriculum, considering the *ethos* of the school, its environment, and social context, to offer to children the necessary knowledge, confidence, and abilities to make choices that promote health.

The concept of Health Promoting Schools (HPS) appeared during the 1980's with WHO support as an integration mechanism of different elements that, in combination, could favour the ultimate success in the attainment of educational and health results [38,53,54] (Box 5.3). These elements would include the curriculum, the school environment, schools services offered by the school, the partnerships with the community, and the school support to health policies.

A Health Promoting School (HPS) can be defined as "a school that constantly strengthens its capacity as a healthy space to live in, to learn, and to work."[55] Its goals of strengthening autonomy over health and structural/environmental action are evident in the development of a series of action programs, which:

- Make efforts to improve the health of school employees, families, and community members, as well as the students'.
- Reinforce health and learning with all available measures.
- Involve health and education workers, teachers, parents, and community leaders in efforts to make the school a healthy environment.
- Make efforts to provide a health environment, school health education, and health services in partnership with community programs, health promotion programs for employees, food and nutrition programs, opportunities for physical education and reestablishment, and counselling, social support, and mental health promotion programs.
- Implement policies and practices that respect individual's self-esteem, promote multiple opportunities for success, and recognize the efforts and positive intentions, as well as personal accomplishments.

This concept of HPS has been spread to several parts of the world as an important strategy that provides opportunities to diminish inequality among youngsters, as well as in the population as a whole.

Evaluations about the impact of this approach have highlighted that the available evidence is limited, but promising.[43,56,57,58] In a systematic review aiming to evaluate the effectiveness of Health Promoting Schools, Lister-Sharp et al.[43] highlight impact evidence of the HPS on the social and physical environment of the school in respect to the development of workers, school food provision, programs of physical exercises, and social relationships, besides improving behavioural aspects linked to health. There is some evidence that this approach can cause positive impacts on aspects of both mental and social health, like self-esteem and violence reduction. They conclude that the most effective results are obtained with several different approaches, combining programmes in the classroom with changes in the school environment and involvement of families and community.

The impact of health promotion in schools was examined by Moysés.[58] Correlating the implementation level of health promotion policies in public schools of peripheral neighbourhoods of Curitiba with the oral health of 12 year-old children. She observed that the schools with the highest level of implementation of health promoting policies (supportive) showed better and more homogenous results, in relation to the percentage of caries-free children and with

Box 5.3 Elements for establishing health promoting schools.

- The curriculum (health contents, educational approach, resources)
- The environment (geographical, psychosocial, physical, and organizational elements of the school and its local community)
- Health services (medical, dental and supporting services at school)
- Community relationships (formal and informal partnerships between school, parents, health sector, and local community)
- School policies (school norms, rules, and practices that maximize the health of the school community)

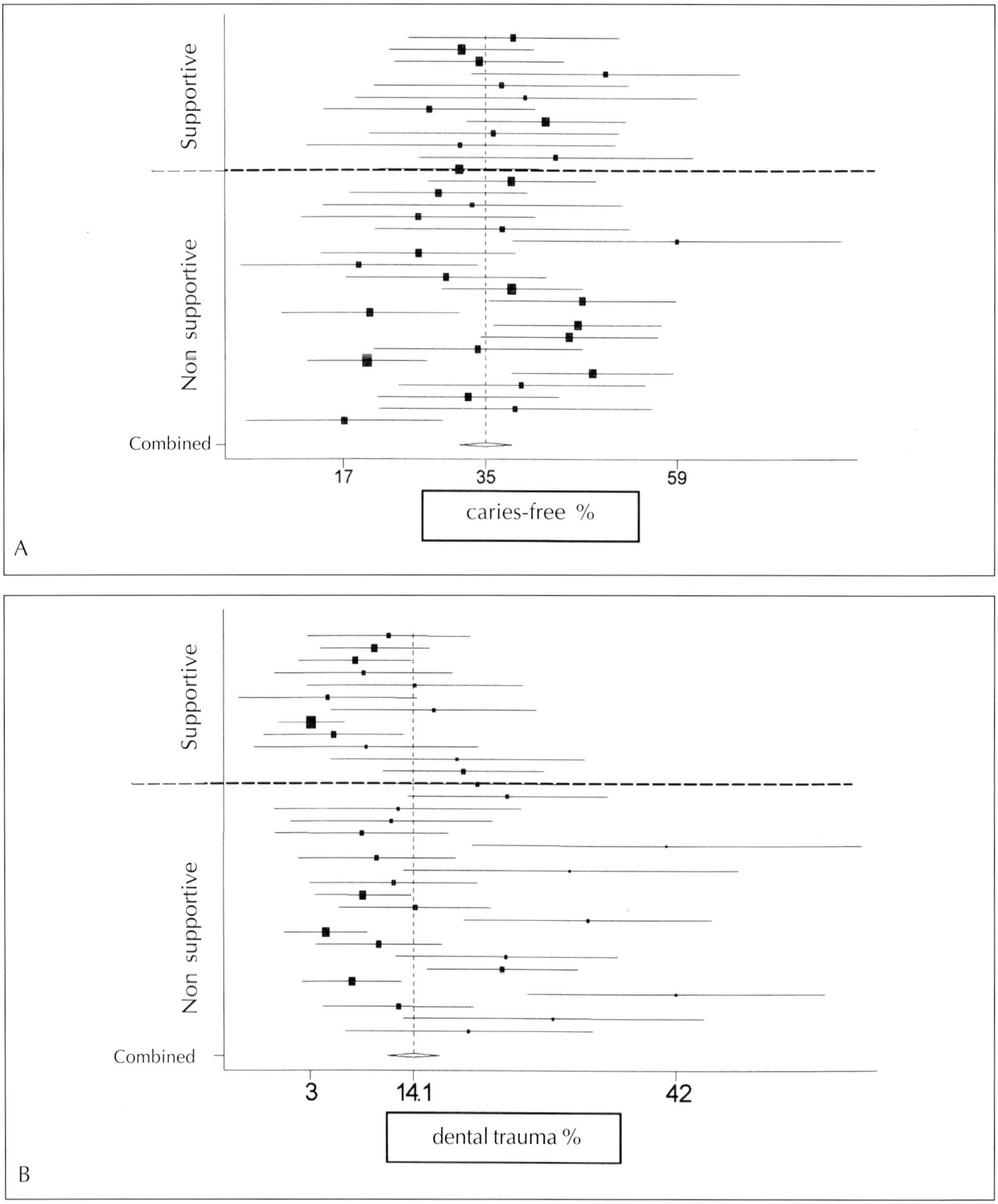

Graph 5.1 A and B Grouped estimation and intervals of confidence by school, according to the level of support to health promotion* and combined estimation obtained by the method of the random effect, for children free from caries and dental trauma.

__ combined estimations

* supportive and non-supportive schools

The rectangles on estimation lines represent the weight given to each school in the calculation of the combined estimation dental trauma than the non-supportive schools, with a lower level of implementation of these policies (Graph 5.1).

More specifically, schools that developed a whole curriculum supported by health policies (fighting smoking and drug use, health nourishment) and centered on the participatory teaching and development of cooperative projects for the improvement of the physical environment of the school, had a higher percentage of caries-free children and less dental trauma. In addition, schools that demonstrated a commitment to health and safety by means of the presence of some responsible for the health promotion at the school, higher involvement of the parents, and development of school safety strategies, had 10% less children with dental trauma than the mean for the control schools (15%). Therefore, health promotion in schools seems to be an important strategy to be developed in collective programmes of oral health promotion for children, making it possible to have a positive impact on health inequalities.

Promoting oral health in Promoting Health Day Care Centres: the significance of a good start

The concern with the education of children under 5 years old is relatively recent, and is linked to the recognition of the rights of both child and woman by society. The day care centre, when appropriately organized, represents an educational space complementary to the family's that favours the physical, cognitive, and affective development of the child, needing an environment that provides conditions for this to happen. The day care centre environment is especially important for the development of health promotion policies in childhood, for some reasons that will be presented here.

Process of expanding of preschool education

General health

In Brazil, as in many other countries, an increasing number of children attend to day care centers.[59] Even though there are concerns related to the prevention of transmissible diseases, especially respiratory infections, [60] the day care centre's environment is considered important for the development of health programmes. Nutritional programmes, for example, are essential for favouring the child's growth and development, especially low income children. Studies about the determination of chronic diseases in adults have reinforced the value of giving priority to health in childhood. According to these studies, diseases originated in the beginning of life and different exposures to cumulative risks during the life course influences chronic disease rates in adulthood.[61]

Oral health

The day care centre environment provides the maintenance of a good oral health for children. Being enrolled in a day care centre results in better oral health, independent of social class and nutritional conditions.[62] A healthy deciduous dentition undoubtedly is an important factor for the development of a satisfactory standard of mastication and speech. Good oral health in childhood prevents unnecessary suffering caused by pain, discomfort, and long treatments.

Acquisition of sustainable behavioural standards

The day care centre environment can also provide the acquisition of healthy behaviours by the child, helping to establish good habits. Diet practices in childhood influence the standard of nourishment choices at later ages, even though the extension of this influence is not well understood.[63,64]

Reduction of social inequalities and its impact on oral health

Preschool education has important effects on health and on children's and families' well being, especially low income children. Apparently, the provision of day care centres seems is an effective policy for fighting poverty, mainly by providing for mothers the possibility of entering the work market.[65,66]

Oral health of children under 5 years old

Dental caries in childhood is still a serious public health problem due to its frequency and for the impact of its consequences on individuals and communities.[14] In Brazil, for children 3 to 6 years of age the caries levels were very high for all ages.[67] Box 5.4 shows the main results of the study in children between 3-6 years old. Other studies in Brazil have confirmed the high prevalence[19,68,69,70] or incidence[71] of caries and the low percentage of children free from the disease at the ages 4-5 years old.[19,69] The high prevalence of caries at childhood is strongly related to socioeconomic factors, more specifically to the excessive intake of sugar and low use of fluoride.[71,72]

Oral health needs in children younger than 5 years of age

The effective provision of health services appropriate to the needs of the population represents a challenge for health planners. Considering the subjectiveness involved in the definition of what is and what is not oral health, and even the limitation of available resources to treat all the sick ones, some authors have defended the adoption of methods that take into account other aspects, beyond the clinical pure evaluation.[73,74,75] A judicious evaluation of the oral health needs, which takes into consideration not only normative needs (clinical ones), but also those perceived by the population, is essential for the establishment of a health promotion project in day care centres environments.

The main reasons for the adoption of wider criteria for the definition of health needs for children under 5 years of age were summarized by Watt:[76]

- To identify oral health determinants.
- To know the concerns of the population.
- To focus on results related to equity.
- To facilitate partnerships.
- To establish initial information for future evaluation.

However, the determination of oral health needs in day care centres demands a certain degree of experience and ability in the use of the indexes. It is advisable to have the participation of an dental public health expert in the project.

Changes in the day care centre environment: the effect of nutritional guidelines

It is important that any strategy of health promotion developed in day care centre environments should be based on scientific evidence. Even though several expert committees from national and international bodies recommend the adoption of guides for the reduction of sugar intake, little research has been conducted to evaluate the effects of these guides. One of these studies measured the effect of the adoption of guides about the increment of dental caries in children enrolled in day care centres of Recife.[71] Results of this work indicated that children enrolled in day care centres that adopted the guidelines for sugar intake consumed less than half of the amount of sugar consumed in day care centres that did not adopted the guidelines: 22.9 g against 53.5 g per day. As a consequence, these children had a 4.9 less chance to develop dental caries when compared to those in day care centres that did not adopt guidelines. The conclusions of the study reinforce the significance of this strategy as an effective way to promote health in the preschool context.

Taking into account consensual recommendations proceeding from expert reports, Watt[76] proposed the following central messages for health promotion activities for children under 5 years old in day care centres environments:

- Sugar intake: the amount and the frequency of non-milk extrinsic sugars must be reduced. Sugared foods and drinks must be restricted to the main meals. The intake of milk, vegetables and fruits must be stimulated.
- Infants' nourishment: maternal milk is the ideal food for babies; however, ideally, sugar must not be added to the weaning diet.
- Drinks: milk and water are the best drinks for children (semi non-fat milk is the best kind of milk after 2 years old, since the child has good nourishment). Non-fat milk, coffee, and black tea are not appropriate for children under 5 years old. Juices containing sugar must be very diluted and consumed only at the main meals.
- Nursing bottles: must be discouraged after 12 months of age. Only milk and water must be served on nursing bottles. Other liquids must be served in glasses.
- Pacifiers: when used, they must not be dived in sugar or sweetened products and they must be disposed before 6 years of age, when the permanent teeth erupt.

The reduction of the excessive consumption of sugars could also be achieved by means of national and local nutrition policies that could give higher incentives to produce and make available healthy foods, regulation of food labels with specifications about the sugar content and composition, withdrawal of non-milk extrinsic sugars (NMES) from pediatric medicines and development of health education programs.

Sheiham[77] highlights that the environment determines the behaviour. So, an effective way of changing the behaviour is to change the environment where people live and are educated. Positive changes in the day care centre environment can influence the decline of dental caries and improve oral cleanliness, and thereby periodontal health, in children

Building the educators' capacity

Another important aspect to oral health promotion in day care centres is building the caretakers' capacity of preschool children caretakers. In the United Kingdom, a document produced by the Health Education Authority,[78] entitled "Smiling for Life", was prepared with the objective of supporting staff and caretakers in the promotion of nutritional and oral healthy practices in day care centres. The document outlines the reasons why caretakers are important:

- Several children spend a significant time receiving care from the day care centre staff.
- They have access to the child when the first teeth erupt, especially those low income ones.
- Caretakers can help parents to transform the family environment in a healthier one for their children.

Most caretakers have no specific education for this kind of work. Caretakers

Chapter 6

Development of Behaviours and Habits Conducive to Oral Health

Claides Abegg

Introduction

Habits and behaviours related to health play an important role on both general and oral health of children and adults. Developing and maintaining them to standards conducive to health will help preserve the individual's health along their life course. This chapter outlines the factors related to the development of behaviours and habits conducive to oral health, and describes the main explanatory factors relating to changing behaviours.

Factors related to the development of behaviours and habits conducive to oral health

Recent theories on human behaviours consider that there are three large groups of factors which influence the development of behaviours and habits conducive to the health of individuals or populations. They are:

- Demographic and social factors – age, socioeconomic status, socialization – influence from social and peer-groups norms, routine nature of several daily life aspects – working and family life, social support.
- Environmental and structural factors – environments that favour or make opportunities to develop or change a behaviour difficult; access to proper resources.
- Psychological factors – models of beliefs in health, self-control on health, self-efficacy.

Demographic and social factors

Sex and socioeconomic status

Differences exist between the sexes in relation to the adoption of preventive habits related to health. Women adopt more health related behaviours and use more medical preventive and therapeutic services than men.[1] Watt and Sheiham,[2] in a study about diet with British adolescents, showed that a higher number of girls compared to the boys tried to reduce the intake of fats. The reason why they tried to change their diet was concern about appearance. Women brush their teeth and use more dental floss more often than men.[3,4,5,6,7,8,9] Possible explanations for these differences between the sexes may be the woman's role with the society, related to socio-cultural and socio-psychological factors,[1] and the pressure that society exerts on women to make them more attractive to men. They are more concerned with the appearance than the boys, and that includes concern about teeth.[10]

The evidence of the association between habits conducive to oral health and socioeconomic status abounds in the literature.[6] There is a social class gradient in oral hygiene habits among people 15 year-old or older. Those in higher compared to lower socioeconomic groups and people who lived in the urban areas rather than rural areas had better habits.[3, 9,11,12] Abegg[7] showed that the social class gradient in oral hygiene persisted into adulthood; higher socioeconomic category brushed their teeth more often and used dental floss more often than lower socioeconomic adults.

Similarly, Watt and Sheiham[2] found differences between adolescents from high and low socioeconomic categories in relation to the change to a healthier diet. Those adolescents from a high socioeconomic category took into consideration educational leaflets about diet, a higher availability of healthy food, and will power. Adolescents from low socioeconomic category did not consider that these factors were important

Social and economic conditions may be facilitators or limit the adoption of habits related to health. The choices' options and the access to information and education of people with low purchasing power are usually more restricted and may make it difficult to adopt behaviours conducive to health. For example, in the case of dental floss use, the economic factor can be a powerful conditioner because it is an expensive item, accessible to a small portion of the population. In the same way, the adoption or the change to healthier diets has cost implications that makes it difficult for low income groups to change their diet.

Socialization

The process of development of attitudes, habits, and behaviours in related to health along the life course is called "health career" or "life course in relation to health".[13] A health career offers to the health professional "the description of the ways by which a person's attitudes develop along the time in relation to health."[14] The main factors that influence over the health career in the different phases of life can be seen in Figure 6.1.[14,15]

The health career begins at childhood. Children learn and adopt behaviours and habits during childhood by the process of socialization. Socialization is a process of transmission of values, such as routines, knowledge , attitudes, considered of significance to survival by people and the community.[13] It is a continuous experience during the whole life. Socialization is usually divided into primary, secondary, and tertiary socialization.[14]

Primary socialization occurs in the beginning of the childhood and it is thought that it is the most important for the human being, considering that it is the period when essential norms and values are applied. In this period, the parents' influence, especially from the mother, on the internalization of the individual's behaviours, attitudes and beliefs is considered the most salient.[16] The primary socialization process happens by means of a system of testing by the child and reward and reprimand and involves modeling. Children identify themselves with the parents' behaviour because that is safest. Good behaviours are rewarded and praised while the "bad" ones can lead to unpleasant reactions. For example, bitter taste is unpleasant to children because bitterness signals poisons. Similarly avoid-

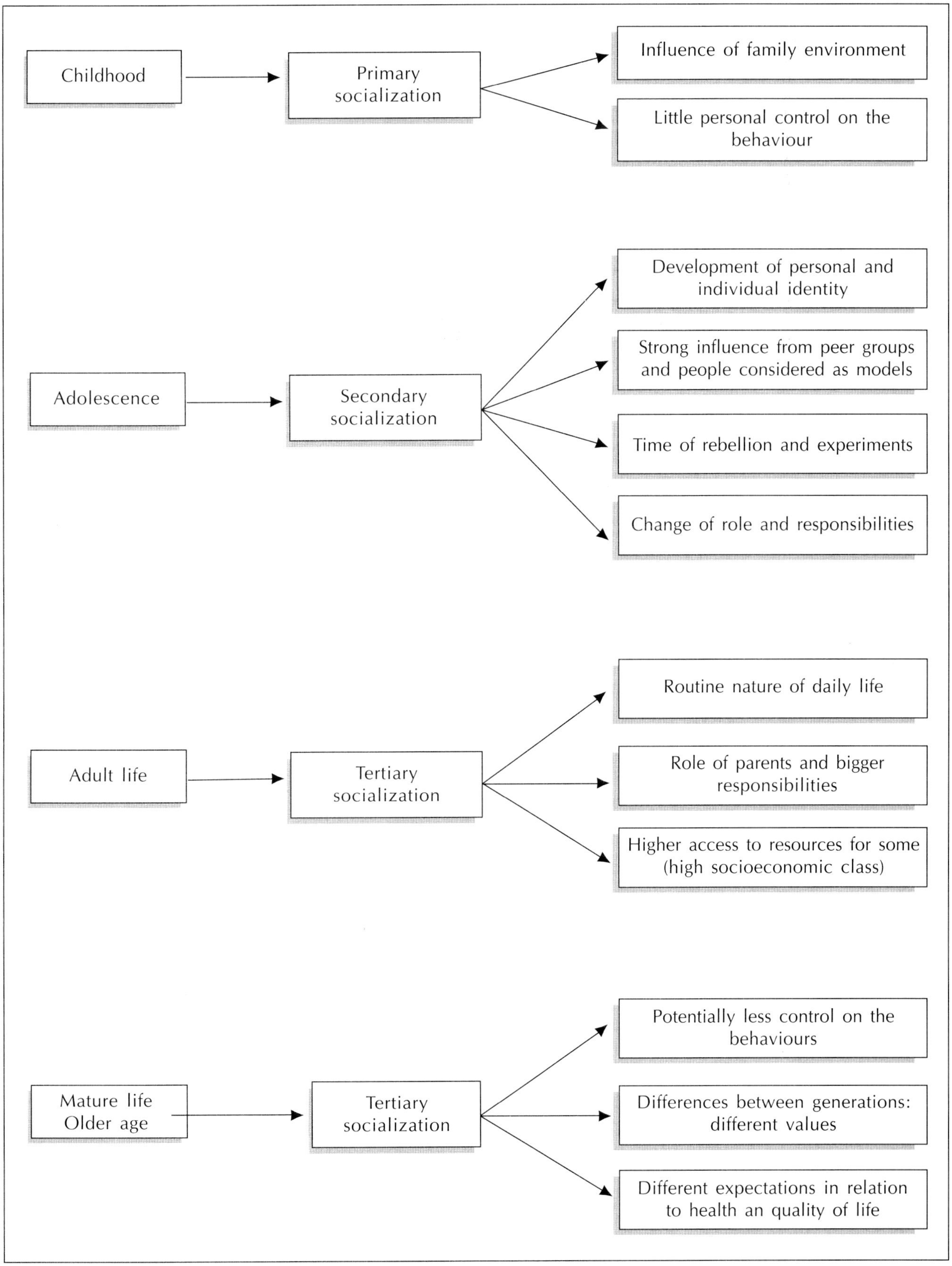

Fig. 6.1 Factors that influence people's behaviour at different stages of life.

ance of dirt and unhygienic products due to their disgusting smell 'teaches' children to avoid such products. In addition, they may be reprimanded and punished. The parents' attitudes and their perception in relation to oral health will influence the child's attitudes and perceptions. A child raised in a family environment where oral health care is not valued will probably become an adult who will not value oral health. Unsurprisingly, oral health and the use of dental services by children are correlated with their mother's.[17] Parents, especially the mother, are the model that children tend to follow by imitating their behaviour. By taking care of children's teeth and body cleaning, parents are showing and teaching the children how they should take care of their teeth and body.[14] This behaviour will be internalized and integrated into daily routines.[18]

Mothers play the central role in the education of very young children in relation to tooth brushing, together with hands and face washing.[16, 19] Children copy their mothers and, by means of this copying, a value is acquired. By reinforcement, this value becomes a habit. In general, children do not like their face, hands and teeth to be washed. This task must be accomplished by the parents.[14] In relation to the child's growth and development of manual dexterity, they will want to wash the body and the teeth in the same way that their parents do. At the end of the first year of life, the majority of the children are being fed with solid foods. Children start the adaptation to the family's dietary standards. It is in this phase that standards of sugar intake are established.[20] Sweet preference is innate because most sweet foods were safe and non-poisonous as well as being highly calorific. Exposing a year old child to much sweetness will alter their taste threshold and they will want sweeter foods in future to satisfy that new threshold.

Secondary socialization merges with primary socialization. The child grows up and establishes relationships outside of the home. Behaviours developed as a result of the primary socialization are influenced and modified by individuals or institutions, such as schools, media, group of friends, colleagues, and other significant people.[13] Quite often, the models that influence the children's behaviour are outside of the family circle at this stage of life. Classroom friends and teachers become models of behaviours in general, as well as of habits related to health.

Groups of friends act either as a positive force or as a strong barrier to preventive behaviours. Adolescents' behaviour in relation to tooth brushing was more susceptible to the group of friends and the influence of relatives than the influence of the dentist.[21] Several studies in schools have shown that the significance of the influence of classroom friends in the development of attitudes and behaviours related to health.[14] In these studies, older children played the role of educators in health, teaching younger children. Gains were obtained in relation to health both for the children playing the educator role and for the ones who were the educating ones.

One of the problems that may occur in this phase of children's life is the conflict that may be established between the health education received in the school and the education at home. This is the reason why the involvement of parents in the health education programmes at school is so significant.

Bateman[23] summarized the factors that influence children on their oral health behaviour during the secondary socialization:

- The continuous influence of parents at home.
- The modeling role of some people, especially artists and other media stars.
- The pressure of the group of friends and school mates to look clean and attractive.

- The advertisement of dental products in the media and the education in general an oral health at schools and by members of the dental staff in clinics and practices.

Beliefs, attitudes, and behaviours that lead to health, learned during the childhood, are important since they are related to health behaviours at the adult age. Besides, when these behaviours are learned early on life, they stay deeply interiorized and resistant to changes.[18]

The media affects secondary socialization and is considered an opinion maker for the population and it plays an important role in attitude formation and behaviours. The media can affect negatively oral health by the promotion of harmful items to general and oral health, like sugary drinks, confections and candies and salty foods, and in general. The positive aspect of the media's role can be observed by the diffusion of the use of toothpaste and toothbrushes. That encourages tooth brushing and improving oral health.[22] At the same time, the increase in the consumption of toothpaste, parallel to the addition of fluoride, had a marked impact on the reduction of dental caries prevalence.[22]

Tertiary socialization occurs in adult life. It is related to the acquisition of new habits and behaviours or changes in the old ones. Tertiary socialization may not happen naturally. This process is influenced by three factors: professionalization, health education, and social norms. Professionalization is associated with the change of values related to the health of people who become health professionals. It is said that in the process of professional education, the person is influenced by other working colleagues. Abilities and the standard of behaviour of acknowledged class mates and teachers are taken as proper by the student. The acquisition of knowledge on the aetiology and prevention of diseases will influence the student.[14] Moreover, the acknowledgement of the health professional by the society as someone who has considerable knowledge on a certain field, provides legitimacy and who gives opinions and counselling on health will influence attitudes and behaviours of the society.

Along the life course, health education is obtained from various sources; school, the work place, and the media can influence attitudes, habits, and behaviours related to a person's health. The third significant aspect in the tertiary socialization is the social norms, whose significance will be discussed below.

Routines

During the socialization process, children learn habits and behaviours that are integrated into daily routines. These habits and behaviours are internalized and are difficult to change in the adult life. The major part of daily activities are inflexible routines.[24] The scenario described by the participants was one of inflexible activities like work, domestic activities, preparation of food and personal hygiene care. Activities associated with getting up and going to bed, such as teeth cleaning and showering, were considered the least flexible ones. [24] The majority of women describe their daily activities as routines.[25] For Graham,[25] considering a context where there are conflicting pressures and little resources, the family's well being may depend on routines by which individual health is shaped. For many families, routines can be considered the choices in relation to health that make their survival possible.

So it clear that habits related to health are integrated in the daily life in a routine way. Due to their routine nature, these habits tend to exist as predictable and relatively stable standards. [26,2] "Health related habits are integrated to social relationships and adaptation processes which are part of a system that is significant for the individual's life."[26]

Confirming the findings for routines in general a dental study with British adults, showed that oral health habits are perceived as part of their daily routines, being accomplished in a sequence of activities, time, and place.[28] Oral hygiene habits are influenced by an interaction of what was learned in childhood and the routine nature at daily life.[28] These routines are based on two important aspects:

- Primary socialization: what was learned as a child. If people had learned how to clean their teeth at a certain time and in a certain place, in association with other activities like washing the face and showering, often this learning was readily kept until the adult life.
- Life style, in which tooth cleaning was integrated to the daily activities of people, and there were competing demands on daily basis, besides a set of social forces like financial limitations, lack of time and energy interfering on the tooth cleaning and reducing its efficiency.[28]

The influence of routine and work on oral health habits was shown by Abegg.[29,30] Those who had less routines and more flexible daily activities showed a higher frequency of tooth brushing. The participants who had more flexibility in their working hours brushed their teeth and used dental floss with a higher frequency, and had a lower dental plaque level.

Structural and environmental factors

A human being's health-related behaviours are also influenced by cultural values and by social forces of the society to which they belong. The human being's tendency is to think that they belong to a certain group or social class. This perception depends on a series of social factors such as occupation, education, income, ethnicity, and race. However, there can be some inconsistency between these factors. When the inconsistency between the social status that the person attributes to herself and what he was able to achieve, he tends to choose the status that provides the higher social status. Once the social status to which the individual believes they belong to is defined, he takes on the habits and behaviours and habits, including those related to health, according to the social structure and the environment where he lives. The Individual is influenced by social values and pressures perceived by him as specific of his socioeconomic category or social class.[19.31]

Social norms play a dominant role on people's behaviours and habits. Social norms are defined as beliefs and values common to the society where the individuals live and interact. These norms define behaviours and habits of a certain society and that are accepted as "normal". Norms provide social cohesion to the group and allow it to have an identity.[18] The influence of values, norms, and social environment that affect habits and behaviours of individuals are relevant to the promotion of a child's oral health, since parents play a fundamental role in the creation of habits conducive to the child's health.

Presently, it is acknowledged that adolescents, especially girls, in industrialized countries, are greatly concerned with their image. The concern with physical appearance may be considered as an important motivating factor in the adoption of and maintenance of oral health preventive habits. Studies accomplished in the USA and Israel showed that adults considered the appearance of the teeth important to make friends and to date. Two thirds of the North-Americans believed that the teeth appearance was an essential factor to get a job.[32]

Among the several factors associated with health-related habits, it is useful to mention the importance of information. The correct information about habits that lead to oral health is essential for oral health promotion. Parents are the main influence in the creation of children's habits that lead to health. Therefore, it is of extreme relevance that they have proper information on aspects related to oral health, like cleaning teeth, proper use of fluoride and about diet, especially regarding sugars intake.

Besides information, it is essential that people's personal means and abilities to adopt health-conducive behaviours are considered. For example, financial resources to buy toothbrushes and toothpastes are essential. The development of the ability to properly use a toothbrush and toothpaste depends mainly on the parents. The recommendations is that they help their children to toothbrush until they are seven years old.

The significance of environments or social spaces supportive to health in the behaviours related to health promotion is widely acknowledged and is discussed in Chapter 5 of this book.

Psychological factors

In the last 20 years, several models involving psychological factors were tested in an effort to understand habits that lead to health promotion. In this section, the most frequently used models will be discussed in relation to oral health promotion.

Health Locus of Control

Health Locus of Control is a derivation of the concept of localized control conceived by Rotter's social learning theory.[33] In this model, we try to understand how much the individuals believe that the events that happen to them, for example, having health or becoming sick, depends on their own efforts and ability, or that they are the result of external factors, such as luck, chance, or destiny. Individuals that believe that they have control over what happens to them are called inners, while those who believe that what happens to them is related to chance or destiny and do not perceive their control over what happens to them are called externals. The external factors have been divided in two dimensions: powerful others' control, when the individual believes that his or her health depends on people with power over his or her life, like doctors and dentists, and those who chance control, related to random factors, to chance.[34]

Odman et al.[35] did not find any significant relationship between the health locus of control and the improvement of abilities in oral hygiene or in the reduction of dental plaque. A study that investigated if the health locus of control would serve to anticipate people's response to a dental plaque control programme concluded that people could be classified into two groups.[36] The first group included individuals who perceived their susceptibility to diseases by influence of strong external factors, or who believed that the susceptibility could be controlled by their own actions. The second group included individuals who considered that the susceptibility to diseases was influenced by luck. The important point is that only the members of the first group had a more positive response to the regimen and plaque control. Children whose mothers had an external control over health showed higher risk of caries when compared to children whose mothers had an internal control of health.[37]

Theory of Reasoned Action

The Theory of Reasoned Action developed by Ajzen and Fishbein[38] postulates that the behaviour is predicted by the intention of the person to accomplish it or not. The intention of adopting certain kind of behaviour is related to two important factors: the subjective norm and the attitude in relation to the behaviour. The subjective norm means that the individuals perceive the desire of other people that they behave in a certain specific way. The attitude is related to the beliefs about the behaviours' consequences, together with the evaluation of the importance of them.[34]

Some applications of the Theory of Reasoned Action have been used on family planning, weight loss, physical exercise, patient's satisfaction, immunization, and hypertension and oral health. Such studies showed that the intention of adopting a certain behaviour always allows previewing its accomplishment, especially when time is short and the intention is clearly defined.[39] In dentistry, the Theory of Reasoned Action has been tested to study the habit of tooth brushing, the intention to use dental floss,[23,40] and search for dental care.[41] In one study, the Theory of Reasoned Action did not explain what affects tooth brushing behaviour.[23] In another study, there was a relationship between intention and behaviour.[40] Overall the Theory of Reasoned Action has been criticized for assuming a simple causal structure, the intention previewing the behaviour, and the attitudes completely mediating the effects of cognition over intention.[34]

Health Belief Model

The Health Belief Model[42,43] considers that the individuals will adopt a preventive behaviour if they feel susceptible to the disease, if the disease is identified as sufficiently severe to affect any aspect of their life style and if they believe that their action can help to overcome the disease or to be more important than any cost involved with it. The initiative to act can be caused by a 'trigger' like the individual perception of the person or by reading about issues related to health.[39] Janz and Becker[43] in a study review about the Health Belief Model and preventive oral behaviours, concluded that for each one of the beliefs in health there was another study or studies that did not achieve the expected correlation. For example, the Health Belief Model was not able to predict the behaviour of children in relation to dental visits,[44] participation in preventive programmes,[45] or the adherence to home mouthwashes.[46,47,48]

There is no consistency in results of empirical studies using the Health Belief Model. On the other hand, the most favourable results are found in retrospective studies, suggesting that, past behaviour predicts the present and future behaviours. Health-related behaviours, such as tooth brushing and dental floss use, are not consequences of beliefs in health. They are most likely to be associated with hygiene and grooming. These habitual behaviours are so automatic that rational considerations on risks and cost/benefit do not modify them.[49]

Self-efficacy

Self-efficacy was initially described by Bandura.[50,51] Since then it has been used in several studies about health-related behaviour. Self-efficacy is the trust that the individual has that a certain behaviour can be adopted or modified, and that he or she can evaluate how much he or she is able to control his or her own behaviour in certain situations.[52]

Self-efficacy sees the change of behaviour as dependent on the ability of the personal perception to deal with stress and annoyance and to mobilize oneself to achieve the proposed objectives. This affects the intention of changing risk behaviours, the effort made to reach that purpose, and the determination to continue trying, in spite of barriers that may undermine the motivation.[53]

Schwarzer,[53] in a review about health behaviours, showed that self-efficacy is a good prognosis of change and of the intention to change behaviour.

- On the intention to use and the real behaviour of dental floss use.
- On the intention of joining to the pre-

vention of the consequences of breast cancer and to the breast self-examination.
- On the intention of using and the use of contraceptives.

Several studies have shown a relationship between self-efficacy and healthy behaviour and it is therefore useful in health promotion.[34]

What changes health-related behaviours?

Health-related behaviours are difficult to modify. Several trials to change oral health-related behaviours by means of health education have been carried out without much long-term success. Health education programmes lead to short term changes in behaviours. However, few long term changes and gains in oral health have been observed.[54,55,56,57] Schou and Locker,[58] in a systematic review about the efficacy of oral health education and promotion programmes, showed that the biggest gains obtained by these programmes were in knowledge and attitudes related to oral health; not in behaviour change

Studies that investigated how people change their behaviours showed that changes in health-related behaviours occur when behaviours integrated into daily routines become conscious over a long period of time. The behaviours become prominent and problematic.[27]

Changes in social relationships favour changes in health-related habits. New friends, a new job, and moving to another address were reasons quoted by people who changed habits like smoking and diet.[27]

The main reasons for changes in oral health habits were being an adolescence, changing working place, making new friends, by suggestion of the dentist, or to give a good example for children.[59] Based on studies that have been investigating changes on health-related behaviours, it can be concluded that:

- The change or acquisition of a new health-related behaviour is difficult to be maintained, unless the behaviour becomes a routine.
- It is easier to make the new activity a routine when it can be integrated into daily activities without representing a big effort and additional cost in time.
- The habit or behaviour needs to become prominent, pointed out, so that its change occurs.
- The prominence of the behaviour needs to appear during a period of time.
- The habit or behaviour cannot be part of the strategies of the individual to deal with difficulties in their life.
- Changes tend to occur when there are changes in the social context in which the person lives, such as family changes, change of work, cultural transition, special training.
- The individual must have social support or sustenance.

Conclusion

Health-related behaviours and habits influence individuals' oral health along life the life course. The behaviours dentists are concerned with are related to diet, cleanliness, risk taking and attitudes to professionals like dentists and doctors. By grouping all these behaviours into dental health behaviours we do a disservice to knowledge about the evolution of behaviours. Each of those behaviours comes from different domains. Diet is obviously related to sustenance. Children at different stages of the life course are either dependent – in first two years when they were traditionally breastfed, – after the age of two children are more 'picky' about what they eat as they must be more cautious about harmful foods. Later they follow what humans are evolved to eat, namely sweet high calorie foods, fats and salt. Fat and salt was rare in the past and highly valued. Sweet preference is instinctive. As regards cleanliness, that behaviour is rooted in concern to avoid infection. All humans clean themselves from when they are physically capable of doing so. Mouth cleaning is part of body cleaning. As shown above, grooming, particularly around puberty, is a universal behaviour, health related but not health directed. Risk taking is important when we consider a neglected aspect of dental public health, namely injuries to teeth. Boys are more risk taking than girls because males need to take risks and show off to attract females. Attitudes to professions will affect dental attendance. These concepts highlight a logical as well as a biological phenomenon. Humans are not empty buckets with blank slates fin their heads. They come into the world with instincts and adaptations to survive and multiply. Socialization depends on a receiver. Nothing comes from nothing. A child is not soft putty that can be molded by their parents and society. A child will respond to stimuli and messages that are conducive to their survival and they are primed to receive. Socialization should be viewed in that light. Primary and secondary socialization occurs during childhood and adolescence, and directly influences the formation of habits and behaviours. In this period, the parents' role is pivotal. At adult life, during the tertiary socialization, a wider range of factors will influence people's habits and behaviours, such as social, environmental, and psychological factors. Indeed their children can influence them. It is the interaction of these factors that determines the health-related behaviours.

Habits and behaviours developed during childhood are deep rooted and are difficult to change in adult age. Changes of health-related behaviours in adult life are associated with changes in the social context in which people live and establish relationships. It is important that individuals have social support or sustenance during the process of change.

The formation of habits and behaviours conducive to health begins in childhood and is essential for both general and oral health of individuals for their whole life. A knowledge of factors that influence them is fundamental for dental professionals, since it is their task to help children and parents and those responsible for planning oral health and health promotion.

References

1. Kandrack MA. Gender differences in health related behaviour: some unanswered questions. *Social Science and Medicine*, 1991; 32:579-90.
2. Watt RG, Sheiham A. Dietary patterns and changes in inner city adolescents. *Journal of Human Nutrition and Dietetics*, 1996;9:451-61.
3. Murtuomaa H. Toothbrushing in Finland. *Community Dent Oral Epidemiol*, 1979; 7:185-90.
4. Nyyssonen V, Honkala E. Toothbrushing frequency in four consecutive studies of Finnish adolescents. *J Clin Periodont*, 1984a; 11:682-8.
5. Nyyssonen V, Honkala E. Oral hygiene status and habitual toothbrushing in children. *Journal of Dentistry for Children*, 1984b; 4:285-8.
6. Gift HC. Current utilization patterns of oral hygiene practices: state-of-the-science review. In: Löe H, Kleinman DV (eds.). *Dental plaque control measures and oral hygiene practices*. Oxford: IRL, 1986; p.39-71.
7. Abegg C. Hábitos de higiene bucal de adultos porto-alegrenses. *Revista de Saúde Pública*, 1997; 31(6): 586-93.
8. Honkala E, Freeman R. Oral higiene behaviour and periodontal status in European adolescents: an overview. *Community Dent Oral Epidemiol*, 1988;16:194-8.
9. Todd J, Lader D. *Adult dental health-dental 1988: United Kingdom*. London: HMSO, 1991.
10. Hodge HC. *Factors associated with tooth-*

brushing behaviour. [Ph.D Thesis], University of Manchester; 1979.

11. Rise J, Haugejorden O, Wold B, Aarö LE. Distribution of dental health behaviours in Nordic schoolchildren. *Community Dent Oral Epidemiol,* 1991a; 19: 9-13.
12. Rise J, Aarö LE. Determinants of dental health behaviours in Nordic schoolchildren. *Community Denti Oral Epidemiol,* 1991b; 19:14-9.
13. Tones BK. Socialisation, Health Career and the Health Education of Schoolchild. *J. Inst Health Educ,* 1979;17(1):23-8.
14. Freeman R. The determinants of dental health attitudes and behaviours. *British Dent J,* 1999;187(1):15-8
15. Croucher R, Watt R. Health Behaviour Change. Comunicação Pessoal. Abegg C. Mestrado em Saúde Pública. Universidade de Londres. 1994.
16. Blinkhorn SA. *Toothbrushing as part of primary socialization.* [PhD Thesis], Manchester, Department of Preventive Dentistry, University of Manchester, 1976.
17. Gift HC. Social factors in oral health promotion. *In:* Schou L, Blinkhorn AS, (eds). *Oral Health Promotion.* Oxford: Oxford Medical Publications, 1993. p.65-98.
18. Baric L, Blinkhorn SA. e MacArthur. A health education approach to nutrition and dental health education. *Health Educat J,* 1974;33:79-90.
19. Rayner JF, Cohen LK. A position on school dental health education. *J Prev Dent,* 1974; 1:11-23.
20. Honkala E. Oral health promotion with children and adolescents. In: Schou, L. and Blinkhorn, A. (eds.). *Oral Health Promotion.* Oxford: Oxford University; 1993. p.169-87
21. Hodge HC, Holloway PJ, Bell CR. Factors associated with toothbrushing behaviour in adolescents. *British Dent J,* 1982; 152:49-51.
22. Downer MC. The role of oral health promotion in oral health policy. In: Schou L, Blinkhorn AS. *Oral Health Promotion.* Oxford: Oxford Medical Publications, 1993. p.121-41.
23. Bateman P. *Understanding and predicting toothbrushing behaviour in adolescents.* MSc. (PhD Thesis) Department of Community Dental Helth, London Hospital Medical College, 1985.
24. Cullen IG, Phelps E. *Diary techniques and problems of urban life.* Joint Unit for Planning Research, University College London, 1975.
25. Graham H. *Women, health and the family.* Brighton: Harvester, 1984.
26. Hunt MS. Macleod, M. Health, behavioural change: some lay perspectives. *Community Medicine,*1987; 9, 68-76.
27. Hunt MS, Martin CJ. Health-related behavioural change – a test of a new model. *Psychology and Health,*1988;2: 209-30.
28. Croucher R. Lay perspectives on oral hygiene performance: their use in hypothesis development. *Community Dent Health,* 1994;11:105-10.
29. Abegg C, Marcenes W, Croucher R. and Sheiham, A. The relationship between tooth cleaning behaviour and flexibility of working time schedule. *J Clin Periodontol,* 1999; 26: 1-5
30. Abegg C, Croucher R, Marcenes WS. Sheiham A. How do routines of daily activities and flexibility of daily activities affect tooth-cleaning behavior? *J of Public Health Dent,* 2000; 154-58
31. Jacob MC, Plamping D. *The practice of primary dental care.* London: Wright, 1989.
32. Silversen J, Kornacki MJ. Controlling dental disease through prevention: individual, institutional and community dimensions. In: Cohen LK, Bryant PS, (eds.). *Social Sciences and Dentistry. A Critical Bibliography.* V.II. London: Quintessence, 1984;p.145-201.
33. Rotter JB, Chance J, Phares EJ. *Applications of a social-learning theory.* New York: Holt, Rinehart and Wiston, 1972.
34. Søgaard AJ. Theories and models of health behaviour. *In:* Schou L, Blinkhorn AS, (eds.) *Oral Health Promotion.* Oxford: Oxford University, 1993; p.25-64.
35. Odman PA, Lange AL, Bakdash MB. Utilization of locus of control in the predictions of patient's oral hygiene performance. *J Clin Periodontology,* 1984; 11,367-72.
36. Galgut PN, Waite IM. Todd-Pokropek A, Barnby GJ. The relationship between the multidimensional health locus of control and the performance of subjects on a preventive peridontal programme. *J Clin Periodont,* 1987;14:171-6.
37. Reisine S, Litt M. Social and psychological theories and their use for dental practice. *Int Dent J,* 1993;43:279-87.

38. Ajzen I, Fishbein M. *Understanding Attitudes and Predicting Social Behavior.* Prentice-Hall, Englewood Cliffs, NJ, 1980.
39. Mullen PD, Hersey JC, Iverson DC. Health behavioural models compared. *Social Science and Medicine,* 1987;24:973-81.
40. McCaul KD, O'Neill HK, Glasgow RE. Predicting the performance of dental hygiene behaviours: an examination of the Fishbein and Ajzen model and self-efficacy expectations. *J Applied Soc Psychol,* 1988;18:114-28.
41. Hoogstraten J, De Haan W, Ter Horst G. Stimulating the demand for dental care: an application of Azjen and Fishbein's theory of reasoned action. *European J Soc Psychol,* 1985;15: 401-14.
42. Haefner DP. The health belief model and preventive dental behaviour. *In*: Becker, M (ed.). *The health belief model and personal health behaviour.* Thorofare: Charles B. Slack, 1974.
43. Janz NK, Becker MH. The Health Belief Model: a decade later. *Health Education Quarterly,* 1984;11:1-47.
44. Kegeles S. Why people seek dental care: a test of a conceptual formulation. *J Human Behavior,* 1963; 4: 166-173.
45. Weisenberg M, Kegeles S, Lünd A. Children's health beliefs and acceptance of a dental preventive activity. *J Health and Social Behavior,* 1980;21:59-74.
46. Kegeles S, Lund AK. Acceptance by children of a daily home mouthrinse program. *Social Science and Medicine,* 1978;12, 199-210.
47. Kegeles S, Lund AK. Adolescent's health beliefs and acceptance of a novel preventive dental activity: replication and extension. *Health Education Quarterly,* 1982;98:192-208.
48. Kegeles S, Lund AK. Adolescent's health beliefs and acceptance of a novel preventive dental activity: a further note. *Social Science and Medicine,* 1984; 19: 978-982.
49. Ingleheart MS, Tedesco LA. The role of the family in preventing oral diseases. In: Cohen LK, Gift HC. (eds.) *Disease Prevention and Oral Health Promotion.* Copenhagen: Munksgaard, 1995; p.271-92.
50. Bandura, A. Self-efficacy: towards a unifying theory of bahaviour change. *Psychological Review,* 1977; 84: 191-215.
51. Bandura A. *Social foundations of thought and action.* Englewood Cliffs: Prentice Hall, 1986.
52. Ogden J. Psycosocial theory and the creation of the risky self. *Social Science and Medicine,* 1995;40:409-15.
53. Schwarzer R. Self-efficacy in the adoption and maitenance of health behaviours: theoretical approaches and a new model. *In*: Schwarzer R, (ed.) *Self efficacy: thought control of action.* Washington: Hemisphere, 1992; p.217-243.
54. Schou, L. Active-involvement principle in dental health education. *Community Dent Oral Epidemiol,* 1985; 13: 128-32.
55. Kiyak HA, Mulligan K. Behavioural research relate to oral hygiene practices: state-of-the-science review. *In:* Löe, H. Kleinman DV, (eds.). *Dental Plaque Control Measures and Oral Hygiene Practices.* Oxford: IRL,1986; p.225-37
57. Kay EJ, Locker D. Is dental health education effective? A systematic review of current evidence. *Community Dent Oral Epidemiol,* 1996; 24:231-35.
58. Schou L, Locker D. A review of the effectiveness of health education and health promotion. *Dutch Centre for Health Promotion and Health Education,* 1994;4: 7-31.
59. Abegg, C. Toothbrushing behaviour and its changes in a group of Brazilian adults (City of Porto Alegre). *In*: Seventy Sixth General Session and Exihbition of the International Association for Dental Research, 1998, Nice. *J Dent Res, 1998;* 77: p.897.

Chapter 7

Healthy Food Policies

Maria do Carmo Matias Freire

Introduction

Food exerts a strong influence on the health of a child. A proper food regimen from birth also has the potential of assuring healthy teeth for life (Fig. 7.1). Dental professionals therefore play a very important role in the promotion of their patients' well being, by promoting healthy food policies. This chapter reviews the effects of nutrition and diet on oral health of children, the context of oral health in global and national nutrition and health scenarios and the promotion of oral health by healthy food public policies.

Nutrition and diet: effects on oral health

Nutrition refers to the intake and absorption of nutrients, while diet refers to the food that is ingested. Both are able to affect the teeth during their formation and by a local direct effect – a post-eruptive effect. That results in:

- Defects on the teeth structure: a purely pre-eruptive effect.
- Dental erosion: a purely post-eruptive effect.
- Dental caries: a pre- and post-eruptive effect.

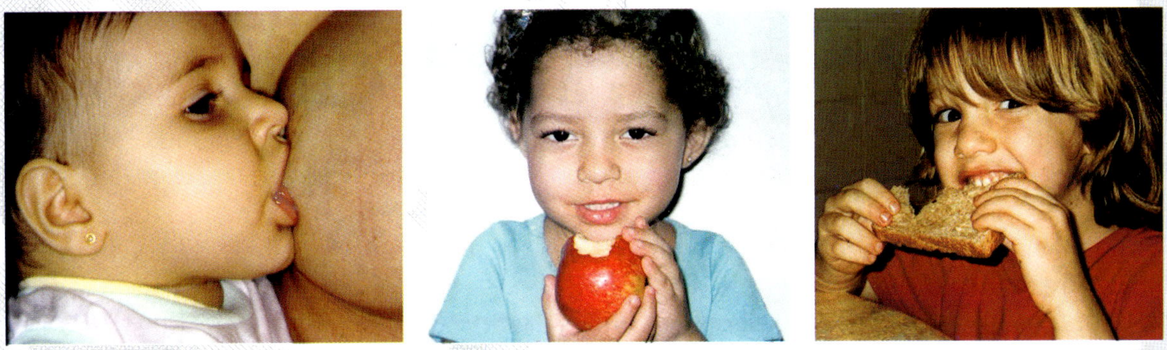

Figs. 7.1 A, B and C Proper nutritional habits are formed in childhood and influence general and the oral health.

Nutritional deficiencies have adverse effects on animals' periodontal tissues, but in humans, the evidence is equivical.[1,2] Only in cases of scurvy (vitamin C deficiency), periodontal tissues of humans are seriously affected, making the inflammatory response to local irritation difficult. However, in general, periodontal tissues benefit from an appropriate nutrition. Diet and nutrition protect against oral cancer particularly from fresh fruits and vegetables.[3,4]

Defects in the structure of teeth

Nutritional deficiency in the period when teeth are formed is one of the causes of defects in their structure. There still is some controversy about the mechanisms by which nutrition affects teeth. The most well known defect is linear enamel hypoplasia, resulting from hypocalcemia.[5] Hypoplasia is common in deciduous incisors of children from developing countries where malnutrition is common, and the hypoplasia can be associated with the development of caries. Another cause of defects in the tooth enamel is the excessive ingestion of fluoride during teeth formation, resulting in fluorosis.

Dental erosion

Diet is the main cause of dental erosion. Erosion is characterized by the loss of dental substance on the oral surfaces of upper incisors. The frequent intake of highly acid solids and liquid foods, mainly soft drinks and manufactured fruit juices, has been the main dietary factor.[6] Soft drinks have a low pH due to the presence of citric or phosphoric acid. In children and adolescents from developed countries, where the intake of soft drinks is very high, soft drinks have been the main cause of dental erosion. Acid juices can also cause erosion. In the deciduous teeth, the risk of erosion is higher when these liquids are administered in nursing bottles. That exposes teeth to acid pH, especially if the nursing bottle is used often to calm the child down.[7] It is possible to substantially reduce the potential erosion by soft drinks and it is hoped that the industry should work to reduce the harm from their products.[8,9]

Dental caries

Pre-eruptive effects

Malnutrition in animals affects dental structure, delays the eruption of teeth and results in an increase in caries. However, the relations are not as clear in humans.[10] It is often difficult to establish if an effect is purely pre-eruptive, since there is the possibility of some post-eruptive influence that cannot be properly separated in observational studies. Longitudinal studies have been problematic in the investigation of the relationship between malnutrition and caries.[10] The best evidence comes from the a longitudinal studies performed in Peruvian children, which show that a moderate to severe episode of malnutrition during the first year of life was associated with increases in caries in both the deciduous and permanent dentition many years later.[11]

Three probable mechanisms explain the relationship between malnutrition and caries: (a) defects in tooth formation; [12-14] (b) delay in tooth eruption; [11,15] and (c) changes in salivary glands.[16, 17]

In countries with appropriate standards of nutrition, the local effect of sugar on the erupted teeth is higher than the pre-eruptive effect. In countries or population groups with severe levels of malnutrition, the pre-eruptive effect can be more important. Malnutrition associated to high intake of sucrose constitutes an important risk factor for the development of caries. Studies performed in low socio-economic population groups in Brazil showed that children with malnutrition had a higher caries index, as well as a higher sugar intake than those without malnutrition.[18, 19]

Post-eruptive effects

The local post-eruptive effect of diet is the main dietary cause of caries.[20] Sugars are the most cariogenic component of diet, acting as a substrate for acid production by plaque bacteria and the subsequent demineralization of dental enamel. Frequency, amount and the kind of sugar ingested influence its cariogenic potential. Sucrose is the most cariogenic sugar, even though glucose, fructose, and maltose shows a cariogenicity that is similar to sucrose. Lactose is the least cariogenic sugar. Starch can cause caries, but much less than sugars. Basic starchy foods, such as rice, potatoes, bread and pasta, are considered a low risk for the child. When refined, cooked and mixed with sugars, such as cookies, breakfast cereals or biscuits, and ingested with some frequency, starch can cause caries. Most caloric sweeteners and all non-caloric sweeteners are non-cariogenic or are of very low cariogenicity. Organic (phytates) and inorganic phosphates can prevent caries in rats, but this effect is lower in humans. Other protective elements of the diet include cheese, proteins, fats and casein, but their practical use is uncertain.

The following classification of sugars, based on their availability to bacteria responsible for caries, has been proposed.[21,22]

- Intracellular or intrinsic sugars: those naturally present in the cell structure of foods, such as fruits and vegetables. They present a very low cariogenic potential and are important for a good nutrition.
- Extra cellular or extrinsic non-lactose sugars: those added to foods, be it by the consumer or by the industry, such as table sugar (usually sucrose), cookies, cakes, soft drinks, manufactured yoghurt, honey and other candies for children. These products, in general, present a high cariogenic potential and deleterious effects when ingested in large amounts.
- Sugar from milk: it is the sugar (lactose) present in milk and its derived. It has a low cariogenic potential and is very important for a good nutrition.

Sugars and caries in children

Most epidemiologic studies show that the caries experience is higher in children with the highest intake of sugar.[23-43] One of the most relevant studies in children – the National Survey on Diet and Nutrition on children from 1.5 to 4.5 years of age in the United Kingdom – showed that the factors most strongly associated to the caries experience were the intake of sugared liquids before going to sleep, the lack of supervision of tooth brushing, family expenditure on sugared candies and the geographic region.[38] Also in the United Kingdom, a ecologic study showed a strong correlation between caries in children between 5 and 12 years of age and the amount of sugar available in the country.[44] The association between sugar consumption and caries in children has been also shown in Brazil.[45-51]

Sugars in children's foods

The problem of high intake of sugars usually starts very early in childhood, with the introduction of sugared foods and drinks in the initial months of life.[38,52-57, 58-60] With this diet, babies develop a preference for sugar which can have an immediate effect on their deciduous teeth and also affects their immediate and future general health, mainly by obesity. Silver [61] observed a correlation between the use of sugared liquids in the nursing bottle at 3 years of age and the intake of sugared snacks later on childhood.

Next, the nourishment in the main periods of childhood will be approached, from birth to approximately 12 years of age, and its effect on the child's oral health. Examples of strategies to improve the child's diet and nutrition, focusing on the reduction of sugars in diet, will also be presented.

Breastfeeding

Exclusive breastfeeding constitutes the ideal diet for the beginning of a child's life, since it is a complete food, protects against infections that are common in childhood, is free from contamination, and the child's metabolism is perfectly adapted to breast milk. During exclusive breastfeeding, there is no need to offer other foods or liquids to the child, not even water, since mother's milk already has it. Millions of children die every year because of diarrhea, respiratory infections and other diseases because they are not properly breastfed.[62,63]

The recommendation of the World Health Organization, dated May 2001, is that the child receives exclusive breastfeeding until six months of age, and that continues to be breastfed until two years of age, receiving food complements from six months of age onwards.[62] This guidance replaces the previous one, which recommended exclusive breastfeeding during the 4 to 6 initial months of age. That was a reason for ambiguous interpretation during several years.

The prevalence of breastfeeding has increased in industrialized countries, but is still below the WHO recommendation.[64] The use of cow's milk is common. Breastfeeding or cows milk without any adding of sugar is not considered cariogenic. The effects of breastfeeding on oral health includes the good development of the masticatory system. Both human and cows milk contain, respectively, 7% and 4.8% of lactose, and has a low cariogenic potential, since lactose is the sugar with the lowest potential to be fermented in acid by dental plaque bacteria.[65-72] Milk also has protective components, such as calcium, phosphorus, antibacterial substances, phosphoproteins (casein), and fats, which help to prevent the enamel dissolution and contribute to its remineralization. The frequency and the length of exposure of the teeth to milk are other important factors in its cariogenicity.

Human milk has a higher proportion of lactose and a lower proportion of calcium, phosphorus and protein than cows milk, but the occurrence of caries in babies due to breastfeeding is very rare.[73] Clinical cases are almost always associated to unrestricted and long lasting nocturnal breastfeeding after teeth eruption, when salivary flow is decreased. During breastfeeding, lips are pressed against the teeth, this way restricting salivary flow and can cause caries, since even in normal conditions this region of the mouth has a low potential to be cleaned by saliva. However, in the case reports, information is usually based on mothers' statements and it does is not always become clear if the child is also taking in other foods containing sucrose or other cariogenic sugars.[56] The early introduction of complementary foods (before six months of age) is a common habit., More than half of the four-month-old breastfed children were receiving complementary foods, including teas and water. [64] Children with caries, regardless of the kind of nursing, showed a higher frequency of daily intake cariogenic foods than caries free children.[74] If the diet of a child is rich in sugar and they are breastfed without any restriction, it can cause caries. Therefore, there is no conclusive scientific evidence that exclusive breastfeeding favours the development of caries.

Feeding with cows milk or powder formulas (cows milk processed by the industry), on the other hand, may represent a risk for children. The percentage of children who use nursing bottles is high, even among breastfed children.[64] Around one third of the children up to one month of life use nursing bottles. This proportion increases to 60% in children between two and seven months of age. In the second year of life, this habit continues in 30% of the children. There is evidence that the cows milk without any sugar added has cariostatic properties.[75] There are few studies about the cariogenicity of formula milks.[76] Several of these products which are sold in the USA show a significant cariogenic potential in animals.[72] In the processing of formula milks, glucose polymers have been added as an energy supplement and there is not enough information about its effect on dental health.[22,77]

Both milk and other liquids with added sugars during its preparation at home or during industrial processing often result in rampant caries, mainly when they are offered before going to sleep.[70,78-82] These liquids are used in teas, fruit juices and cool drinks, and sugared soft drinks.[55,83-85] In many countries adding other ingredients to milk, like chocolate, coffee, honey and flours, besides sugar, is very common.[59,86-90] There is evidence that fruit juices are cariogenic,[78] but it is still not clear if this cariogenicity depends on the presence of added sugar, on the absence of salivary stimulation from the fibre components of the fruit, or if the crushing of sugar, making them extrinsic to the cells of the fruit during the extraction of liquid, makes it more cariogenic.[91]

The effect of breastfeeding or the nursing bottle should not be taken in isolation. Studies have shown that the low socioeconomic status has an influence on the development of caries at early childhood[92,93] and it constitutes a strong factor than the kind of nursing.[94] Nutritional deficiency in the prenatal period can cause defects in enamel, predisposing teeth to caries.[94,95]

Complementary nourishment

This period, wrongly named "weaning", should be started from six months of age onwards, with the expansion of the diet to include other solid and liquid foods, besides milk.[56,95] The aim is to reach a diet that will satisfy the nutritional needs for the child's growth and well-being. When feeding practices are introduced to the child varies according to the socioeconomic status and culture. Usually the mother has a higher influence on the choice of foods offered to her children in this period and depend on health professionals for support.[52] The role of the parents in the formation of the child's habits is discussed on Chapter 6. The eruption of the first teeth usually coincides or starts with the complementary nourishment and, therefore, the composition of diet is fundamental to dental health.

WHO Nutrition Department, concerned with the problem of caloric deficiency that torments poor countries, recommends that sugars and honey should be added in small amounts to foods.[96] In Europe, the maximum recommended intake of extrinsic sugars for young children is 10% of the total energy.[97-99] The Health Department of the United Kingdom [97] recommends that, in complemen-

sold had a lower incidence of caries within a two-year period, when compared to children from school that sold candies.[119,120] In English schools, a relationship between the sales of cookies and caries experience in incisors was found.[121]

In most countries, institutional school meals are usually rich in sugars.[122-124] Besides that, students have access to other industrialized or non-industrialized sugared products that are sold inside the schools or in their surroundings. Often they consume them during classes as well. In private schools, the existence of commercial canteens without any systematic guidance in relation to the nutritional quality of foods, selling products with a low nutritional value, rich in sugars, salt and fats, promoted by television advertisements, is common.[125-128] The regulation of these products' advertisement, especially those messages directed toward the children audience, is an important strategy to be developed.

The decentralization of school nutrition programmes offers a good opportunity to improve the quality of the nourishment provided to students from public schools, making it possible to the use of natural (not industrially processed) and regional foods, replacing the pre-prepared industrialized products, usually rich in sugar. [118,129]

Sugars in children's medicines

Besides foods, a great number of oral medicines for children contain sugars, aiming to make them more palatable. A high concentration of sucrose has been found in several kinds of children's medicines,[130] syrups, lozenges for sore throat, and homeopathic globules.[132] However, information on the kind and amount of sugar contained in medicines usually are not available to the consumer.

Medicines containing sugars can cause caries when used several times a day and mainly at night, for long periods of time for treatment of chronic diseases. The presence of caries in some groups of children with chronic diseases, such as brain palsy, epilepsy, mental delay, haemophilia, and heart, renal and respiratory problems, may put their health or even their lives at risk, as a direct result of the disease or the dental treatment .[133]

Sugared medicines in the form of liquids or syrups cause a pH drop in the plaque which is equal or higher than the one caused by a sucrose solution[134] and by similar non-sugared medicines.[131,135,136,137] In the United Kingdom and in the USA, children who used to ingest sugared medicines for a long period had a higher caries experience than control groups.[138-140]

Control measures for the use of sugared medicines by children are necessary and can be integrated into the national policy on medicines.[141] The following actions have been recommended in developed countries, involving the participation of several sectors, such as the consumers, the professionals who prescribe them, the people who dispense them, those involved in the processing, trading, distribution, and sales of medicines, as well as universities, institutes of research, non-governmental organizations, and professional associations.[133,142-145]

- Reformulation of the composition of paediatric medicines in the form of liquids and syrups by not using sugar or using other non-cariogenic sweetener substances.
- Health education for health providers, pharmacists, and parents about the risks of sugared medicines.
- Use of labels in all medicines, containing a complete list of its components and, if there is sugar in the composition, its kind and concentration should

be informed both in the label and in the information sheet.

- Incentives to doctors to prescribe sugarless medicines whenever they are available. As an alternative, pills can be prescribed, which can be crushed and ingested in non-sugared liquids or foods.
- Use of other methods of administering medicines, such as the rectal, intramuscular, inhalation, and transdermal ways.

Because of pressure from medical and dental groups, the pharmaceutical industry has already developed alternative formulas without sugar or with alternative sweeteners, and lists of liquid sugarless medicines are available to health professionals in those countries. The use of pills instead of liquids has been well accepted among parents, health professionals, and teachers, being considered easier to administer.[144] Oral health professionals play an important role in this process, involving themselves in groups that promote such policies, as well as raising awareness of parents about the ways to decrease the caries risk in child patients who use sugared medicines for long periods of time.[133]

Oral health and nutrition in a general health context

Global and national scenarios of nutrition and health

Rapid changes in diets and lifestyles resulting from the industrialization, urbanization, economic development, and globalization of the market, are causing significant impacts on the nutritional status of populations.[146] Parallel to malnutrition, obesity is nowadays one of the most visible problems of public health and, at the same time, the most neglected. According to the World Health Organization, an increasing global epidemic of overweight and obesity has occurred in both developed and developing countries and, if immediate actions are not implemented, millions of people will suffer a range of serious health problems.[147] Obesity is, in general, caused by excess of calories in the diet, mainly from fats and sugars, and lack of physical exercise.

Obesity contributes for the development of many chronic diseases, including diabetes, hypertension, stroke, cardiovascular diseases, and some kinds of cancer. There is considerable evidence relating diets to a high content of sugar to these diseases, besides dental caries, gallbladder stones, gastrointestinal problems, micronutrients deficiency, bone loss, and bone fracture.[4, 21,148,149] The progressive increase of chronic diseases calls also calls attention to the excess in the children's nourishment during the initial years of life.[56, 150] The prevention of chronic diseases must begin during the childhood with health nourishing habits. Children's obesity is an important predictor to adult obesity. Around one third of obese preschool and half of school children become obese adults. Besides that, obesity affects the health of the child, increasing the risk of hyperlipidemia, hypertension, and abnormal intolerance to insulin.[151]

Data about the nutritional state and the nutritional intake of some populations are show that the situation has substantially changed from the 1960's.[152,153,154] The traditional diet, based on cereals, legumes, and other vegetables, has been gradually replaced by processed or semi-processed foods of low nutritional value, promoted by the media as a symbol of high social status. Consequently there has been an increase in the obesity among adults from all economic layers, especially in low income families. In Brazil, the indexes of obesity

Box 7.2 Prevalence of malnutrition and obesity in Brazilian children from 1 to 4 years of age, by *per capita* family income.[154]

Family income layers	1974/75		1989	
	Malnutrition	Obesity	Malnutrition	Obesity
30% poor	26,5	3,8	12,2	2,5
40% intermediate	11,6	4,5	3,8	4,9
30% rich	3,9	9,0	1,4	10,6

are also increasing in children and they have been more elevated in the groups with the highest family income (Box 7.2).[154] In the past decades, there has been an increase in the prevalence of chronic diseases related to the diet, and cardiovascular diseases and cancer are nowadays the main causes of mortality by disease in the Brazilian adult population.[155]

The amount of available sucrose in countries like Brazil is around 55 kg/person/year.[156] This is much higher than the acceptable levels for a good oral and general health: 15 kg in fluoridated regions and 10 kg in non-fluoridated regions.[157] In relation to the relative contribution to the total caloric intake, sugar was about 14.5% in 1988,[158] while the maximum recommended by the WHO is 10%.[159]

In spite of the recent reports of caries decrease in Brazilian children, groups from a lower socioeconomic level still have a high caries experience.[160-163] This tendency is also observed on preschool children.[93] In these groups, which usually have little access to fluoride, poor oral hygiene and a low level of information, diet constitutes an important risk factor. The epidemiology of dental caries in Brazil is discussed in Chapter 1.

The nutritional and oral health picture in many countries shows there is a need for public diet and nutrition policies for the population.

Public policies on diet and nutrition

Developing countries have a great challenge to implement public policies that make it easier to adopt healthy diet and nutrition habits that, at the same time, contribute to the decrease of chronic diseases, nutritional deficiencies and infectious diseases.[164,165]

The present recommendation for a healthy diet are compatible with those suggested to maintain oral health and includes the reduction in the intake of sugars and their replacement with healthy foods that are energy sources as well. Foods like fruit, vegetables, and cereals. In practice, these goals are not easily reached by the population. In the case of sugar, there is strong pressure on the part of sugar and drinks industry, which extols the virtues of sugars.

It is necessary to develop ways to raise awareness of both professionals and the public about the importance of diet for good health, including oral health. Health education constitutes an important measure in this process. Even though the individual counseling for each patient is not realistic and often results in only temporary changes,[166] some children can be benefit if their parents receive the necessary information. Broader measures are needed so that changes in the population can be achieved.

The concept of health promotion includes the development of means that allow the community or an individual to improve and exert a higher control on their health.[167] In this sense, health education must be integrated to a wider policy, able to intervene on the real determinants of the health-disease process and providing to the population not only the necessary information for change but to the healthier options as well. Oral health promotion must, therefore, be integrated into the general health policies and be supported by the principle of the common risk factor, since the intake of sugar is as an aetiologic factor of caries as much as for other chronic disease.[168,169] The dietary recommendations for the prevention of caries coincide with those aimed not only for the prevention of diseases, but for general health maintenance as well. Several health promotion actions must occur at the central level, by means of national policies; others at the community or local level, while others are more appropriate at the individual level. The important thing is that at all levels there is consistency in the information about diet and health. Consensus is crucial in this process, since conflicting messages or recommendations confuse the public and undermines their trust in professionals.

There has been little progress on public diet and nutrition policies in relation to dental public health in the way suggested in this chapter. In the past years, some municipalities have developed local strategies trying to make access to healthy diets easy. For example one city developed the "People's Big Market," a trading programme of locally produced agricultural-farming goods at a low cost (up to 30% less expensive) for low income populations, besides offering educative activities about nutrition and health.[170] Another city government implemented the "Municipal Nutrition Bank," which aims to collect good food to be consumed, but that for some reason could not be traded. The donations are by commercial and industrial establishments and collaborators. They provide foods or meals to assist institutions that distribute them among needy families.[171]

With the increasing interest on health promotion, dentists are being motivated to play a more active role in promoting people's health, acting jointly with other professionals from the fields of health and education and social services (see Chapters 9 and 10). It is necessary to act in an inter-sectoral way on actions that decrease social inequality, improve information, stimulate healthy practices with local resources, and promote improvements both in the oral health and general health of the population. The planning of chronic diseases prevention actions does not only involve health policies, but finance, agriculture, industry, employment, development, trading and education policies as well.[165]

In relation to the policy to decrease sugar intake, Sanderson[172-173] proposed that such a policy must not be based only on educative strategies, but it must include other strategies as well; policies such as regulation, replacement, and strategy on pricing directed towards the several sectors involved; from the production to the final consumer of sugar. The food chain includes producers, refiners, brokers, distributors, providers, consumers, pressure groups, health professionals and public institutions (Box 7.3). In this model, the cooperation between several governmental institutions is essential. No matter what strategy has been chosen, it is advisable to gradually introduce it in order to avoid a confrontation with consumer preferences and giving time for industry to adapt.

Nutritional guidelines and healthy nutritional

Authoritative and non commercial nutritional guides and guidelines are extremely useful to inform national policies, community efforts and individual action. These documents are common in Europe and the USA. They include several aspects of nutrition, diet and health, and conclude with dietary recommendations aiming to prevent health problems that result from nutritional excess. They are often elaborated by government institutions, like health ministries or national departments, or by other na-

genicidade e propriedades cariostáticas por diferentes tipos de leite: revisão. *Arch Latinoam Nutr,* 2000, jun; 50(2):113-20.

77. Moynihan PJ, Gould MEL, Huntley N, Thorman S. Effect of glucose polymers in water, milk and a milk substitute on plaque pH *in vitro. Int J Paediatr Dent,* 1996;6:19-24.
78. Winter GB. Problems involved with the use of comforters. *Int Dent J,* 1980;30:28-38.
79. Dilley GJ, Dilley DH, Machen J. Prolonged nursing habit: a profile of patients and their families. *J Dent Child* 1980;47(2):29-31.
80. Johnsen DC. Characteristics and backgrounds of children with "nursing caries". *Pediatr Dent,* 1982;4:218-21.
81. González-Pérez S, Ventura-Juárez J, Campos-Rodríguez P. Estudio sobre prevalencia de caries dental y caries rampante en población preescolar. *Bol Med Hosp Infant Mex,* 1992;49(11):750-6.
82. Douglass JM, Tinanoff N, Tang JM, Altman DS. Dental caries patterns and oral health behaviors in Arizona infants and toddlers. *Community Dent Oral Epidemiol,* 2001 Feb; 29(1):14-22.
83. Palmer JD. Dietary habits at bedtime in relation to dental caries in children. *Br Dent J,* 1971, Apr;130:288-93.
84. Duggal MS, Curzon MEJ. An evaluation of the cariogenic potential of baby and infant fruit drinks. *Br Dent J,* 1989;166: 327-30.
85. Nacao M, Chuan LP, Rodrigues CRMD. Análise dos hábitos de dieta em crianças por meio da utilização de diários alimentares. *Rev Odontol Univ São Paulo,* 1996 out/dez; 10(4):275-80.
86. Gomes MP, Souza IPR, Modesto A, Ruschel HC. Fatores envolvidos no desenvolvimento da cárie de amamentação. *Rev Assoc Paul Cir Dent,* 1996, nov/dez; 50(6):497-501.
87. Saito SK, Deccico HMU, Santos MN. Efeito da prática de alimentação infantil e de fatores asociados sobre a ocorrência da cárie dental em pré-escolares de 18 a 48 meses. *Rev Odontol Univ São Paulo* 1999 jan/mar;13(1):5-11.
88. Oliveira FC, Long SM, Chelotti A. Avaliação dos hábitos alimentares e de hygiene bucal e sua relação com os índices de cárie e placa, em crianças de 3 a 5 anos de idade de instituições públicas de ensino da cidade de Vinhedo-SP. *Rev Paul Odontol,* 2001, nov/dez;23(6):29-32.
89. Dini EL, Holt RD, Bedi R. Caries and its association with infant feeding and oral health-related behaviours in 3-4-year-old Brazilian children. *Community Dent Oral Epidemiol,* 2000;28:241-8.
90. Nelson-Filho P, Queiroz AM, Mussolino ZM, Assed S. Avaliação dos hábitos alimentares em crianças portadoras de cárie de mamadeira. *J Bras Odontopediatr Odontol Bebê,* 2001, jan/fev;4(17):30-5.
91. Rugg-Gunn AJ. Nutrition, diet and dental public health. *Community Dent Health* 1993;10(Suppl 2):47-56.
92. Ismail AI. Prevention of early childhood caries. *Community Dent Oral Epidemiol* 1998; 26(suppl 1):49-61.
93. Freire MCM. Prevalência de cárie e fatores socioeconômicos em pré-escolares: revisão da literatura. *Rev Bras Odontol Saúde Coletiva,* 2000, jan/jun 1(1):43-9.
94. Smith PJ, Moffatt ME. Baby-bottle tooth decay: are we on the right track? *Int J Circumpolar Health,* 1998; 57(suppl 1): 155-62.
95. Davies GN. Early childhood caries: a synopsis. *Community Dent Oral Epidemiol,* 1998;26(suppl 1):106-16.
96. World Health Organization. Department of Nutrition for Health and Development. *Complementary feeding: family foods for breastfed children.* Geneva: WHO; 2000.
97. Department of Health. *Weaning and the weaning diet. Report of the Working Group on the Weaning Diet of the Committee on Medical Aspects of Food Policy.* London: HMSO; 1994. Report on Health and Social Subjects 45.
98. Holt RD, Moyhihan PJ. The weaning diet and dental health. *Br Dent J,* 1996, Oct 5; 181(7):254-9.
99. World Health Organization. *Feeding and nutrition of infants and young children: guidelines for the WHO European Region, with emphasis on the former Soviet countries.* Copenhagen: WHO Regional Office for Europe;2000. WHO Regional Publications, European Series, 87.
100. Ministério da Saúde. *Estudo qualitativo nacional sobre práticas alimentares;* 1998.
101. Birkhed D. Sugar content, acidity and effect on plaque pH of fruit juices, fruit drinks, carbonated beverages and sport drinks. *Caries Res,* 1984; 18(2):120-7.
102. Grobler SR, Jenkins GN, Kotze D. The effects of the composition and method of drinking of soft drinks on plaque pH. *Br Dent J,* 1985;158:293-6.
103. Amato D, Maravilla A, García-Contreras F, Paniagua R. Los refrescos y la salud. *Rev*

Invest Clin, 1997, Sep-Oct;49(5):387-95.
104. Guthrie JF, Morton JF. Food sources of added sweeteners in the diets of Americans. *J Am Diet Assoc*, 2000; 100:43-8.
105. Ministério da Saúde. Instituto Nacional de Alimentação e Nutrição. *Estudo multicêntrico sobre consumo de alimentos: relatório final*. Campinas: UNICAMP/ UERJ; 1997.
106. Egashira EM, Philippi ST, Monteiro CA, Latorre MRDO. Diet's characteristics for children under two years of age in the city of São Paulo-Brazil. *In: Anais da XXXVI Reunião da Sociedade Latino Americana de Investigação Pediátrica*; 1998 Nov; São Pedro, São Paulo, Brazil; 1998. p.47.
107. Sanderson ME, Winkler JT. *A research report on the labelling of sugars in manufactured foods*. London: Action & Information on Sugars; 1989.
108. Tyrrel A, Rugg-Gunn A. A survey of nutrition labeling of sugar-containing foods in the north of England in 1989. *Community Dent Health*, 1990, Mar; 7:359-67.
109. ANVISA. *Resolução – RDC nº 40, de 21 de março de 2001*. Disponível em: URL:http://www.anvisa.gov.br/legis/resol/40 01rdc.htm [2002 Jun 17].
110. Durward L, Cox S, Freeman R. *Sugar in baby foods*. London: The Maternity Alliance; 1988.
111. Watt R, Fuller S. Approaches in oral health promotion. In: Pine CM, editor. *Community Oral Health*. Oxford: Wright; 1997. p.238-51.
112. Rugg-Gunn A. Nutrition, dietary guidelines and food policy in oral health. In: Pine CM, editor. *Community Oral Health*. Oxford: Wright; 1997. p.206-20.
113. Caroline Walker Trust. *Eating well for under-five years in child care: practical and nutritional guidelines*, Report of an expert working group. London: CWT; 1997.
114. Rodrigues CS. Guia alimentar e incidência de cárie dentária em crianças matriculadas em creches públicas do Recife, Brasil. *Rev Fac Odontol UPE* 1999; 17(1):11-8.
115. Rodrigues CS, Sheiham A. The relationships between dietary guidelines, sugar intake and caries in primary teeth in low income Brazilian 3-year-olds: a longitudinal study. *Int J Paediatr Dent*, 2000;10:47-55.
116. Harris R. Biology of the children of Hopewood House, Bowral, Australia. 4. Observations on dental caries experience extending over 5 years (1957-61). *J Dent Res*, 1963;42:1387-99.
117. Silverstein SJ, Knapp JF, Kircos L, Edwards H. Dental caries prevalence in children with a diet free of refined sugar. *Am J Publ Hlth*, 1983;73:1196-9.
118. Costa EQ, Ribeiro VMB, Ribeiro ECO. Programa de alimentação escolar: espaço de aprendizagem e produção de conhecimento. *Rev Nutr Campinas* ,2001, set/dez; 14(3):225-9.
119. Fanning EA, Gotjamanos T, Vowles NJ. Dental caries in children related to availability of sweets at school canteens. *Med J Austr*, 1969; i: 1131-2.
120. Roder DM. The association between dental caries and the availability of sweets in South Australian school canteens. *Austr Dent J*, 1973;18:174-82.
121. Pengelly JPB, Smith FJA. Incisor caries and primary schools tuckshops. *Publ Health London*, 1972;86:183-8.
122. Quelhas MCP. *Análise da merenda escolar oferecida aos alunos do pré-escolar e escolar pela Secretaria Municipal de Educação de Niterói - RJ* [dissertação]. Rio de Janeiro: Universidade Federal Fluminense; 1988.
123. Barberato MAC, Toledo OA. Cariogenicidade da merenda escolar. *Rev Gaúcha Odontol*, 1991, mar/abr; 39(2): 127-33.
124. Coelho DT, Damiani CR, Gomes JC, Bicudo MH. Avaliação nutricional e aceitabilidade de alimentos formulados utilizados em programas institucionais. *Semina* 1991;11(2):97-101.
125. Silva MV, Pipitone MAP. Cantinas escolares e merenda escolar: convivência possível? *Rev Bras Saúde Esc*, 1994; 3(1-4):23-31.
126. Vilaça EL, Paixão HH, Pordeus IA. A mídia e as tendências de consumo de produtos contendo sacarose por crianças e adolescentes. *Arquivos Odontol*, 1997, jan/jun; 33(1):15-24.
127. Mainardi APR, Oliveira MDM, Finger AT, Pinto AS, Leonardelli A, Dariva C et al. Influência dos comerciais da televisão nos hábitos dietéticos. *Rev Fac Odontol Univ Passo Fundo*, 1998, jan/jun;3(1): 35-40.
128. Wilson N, Quigley R, Mansoor O. Food ads on TV: a health hazard for children? *Aust N Z J Public Health*, 1999, Dec; 23(6): 647-50.
129. FNDE. *Programa Nacional de Alimentação Escolar*. Disponível em: URL:http://www.fnde.gov.br/programas/pnae/index.htm [2002 jun 16]

130. Novais SMA, Grinfeld S, Santana MLA, Almeida IP, Barreto VR, Santos VIM. Cariogenicidade de medicamentos em crianças na faixa etária entre 0 e 6 anos de idade. *Rev Fac Odontol Univ Fed Pernamb,* 1998;8(2):104-9.
131. Neiva A, Silva VS, Maia LC, Soares EL, Trugo LC. Análise *in vitro* da concentração de sacarose e pH de antibacterianos de uso pediátrico. *Pesq Bras Odontop Clin Integr* 2001, jan/abr;1(1):9-16.
132. Koo MH, Cury JA. Concentração e tipos de açúcares presentes em produtos alimentícios, guloseimas e medicamentos encontrados no mercado brasileiro. *Rev ABO Nac* 1996, jun/jul;1(3):172-5.
133. Hobson P. The effects of sugar-based medicines on the dental health of sick children. *Br Dent J,* 1984;8:155-6.
134. Feigal RJ, Jensen ME, Mensing CA. Dental caries potential of liquid medications. *Pediatrics* 1981, Sep;68(3):416-9.
135. Rekola M. *In vivo* acid production from medicines in syrup form. *Caries Res,* 1989;23:412-6.
136. Marathaki E, Pollard MA, Curzon MEJ. The effect of sucrose in medicines on plaque pH. *Int J Paediatr Dent,* 1995;5:231-5.
137. Silva MFA, Guimarães JATL. Potencial cariogênico de medicamentos utilizados no tratamento de doenças do trato respiratório e alergia. *J Bras Odontopediatr Odontol Bebê,* 2001, set/out;4(21):383-6.
138. Roberts IF, Roberts GJ. Relation between medicines sweetened with sucrose and dental disease. *Br Med J* 1979, jul;7; 2(6181):14-6.
139. Feigal RJ, Gleeson MC, Beckman TM. Dental caries related to liquid medication intake in young cardiac patients. *J Dent Child,* 1984, Sep/oct;51(5):360-2.
140. Maguire A, Rugg-Gunn AJ, Butler TJ. Dental health of children taking antimicrobial liquid oral medication long-term. *Caries Res,* 1996;30(1):16-21.
141. Romano-Lieber NS. Política de medicamentos. *Mundo Saúde* 2000 jan/fev;24(1):45-50.
142. Dangor CM, Veltman AM. Sugar-free liquid pharmaceuticals. *S Afr Med J,* 1986;Aug 16;70(4):199-200.
143. Shaw L, Glenwright HD. The role of medications in dental caries formation: need for sugar-free medication for children. *Pediatrician,* 1989;16(3-4):153-5.
144. Manley MC, Calnan M, Sheiham A. A spoonful of sugar helps the medicine go down? Perspectives on the use of sugar in children's medicines. *Soc Sci Med,* 1994; sep;39(6):833-40.
145. World Health Organization. *Report of the WHO expert committee on national drug policies – Contribution to updating the WHO guidelines for developing national drug policies.* Genebra: Action Programme on Essential Drugs/WHO; 1995.
146. Drewnowski A, Popkin BM. The nutrition transition: new trends in the global diet. *Nutr Rev,* 1997;55:31-43.
147. World Health Organization. *Nutrition.* Available from: URL:http://www.who.int/nut/htm [2001 Nov 15].
148. Food and Agriculture Organization/World Health Organization. *Carbohydrates in human nutrition.* Rome: FAO/WHO; 1998.
149. United States Department of Agriculture and United States Department of Health and Human Services. *Dietary guidelines for Americans 2000,* 5th ed. Home and Garden Bulletin No. 232. U.S. Washington (DC): Government Printing Office; 2000.
150. World Health Organization. *Prevention in childhood and youth of adult cardiovascular diseases: time for action.* Report of a WHO Expert Committee. Geneva: WHO; 1990. Technical Report Series 792.
151. Martorell R. Obesity. *In*: Flores R, Gillespie S. *Health and nutrition: emerging and reemerging issues in developing countries.* Washington: International Food Policy Research Institute/2020 Vision; Feb 2001. Focus 5. Brief 7.
152. Leal MC, Bittencourt SA. Informações nutricionais: o que se tem no país? *Cad Saúde Pública* 1997, jul/set;13(3):551-5.
153. Monteiro CA, Mondini L, Medeiros de Souza AL, Popkin BM. The nutrition transition in Brazil. *Eur J Clin Nutr* 1995; 49:105-13.
154. Monteiro CA, Mondini L, Medeiros de Souza AL, Popkin BM. Da desnutrição para a obesidade: a transição nutricional no Brasil. *In:* Monteiro CA. *Velhos e novos males da saúde no Brasil: a evolução do país e suas doenças.* São Paulo, HUCITEC/NUPENS/USP; 2000.
155. Ministério da Saúde. *Mortalidade proporcional por grupos de causas.* Disponível em: URL:http://www.datasus.gov.br/cgi/tabcgi [2001 Jan 5].
156. International Sugar Organization. *World* per capita *consumption of centrifugal sugar.* London: ISO; 1999.
157. Sheiham A. Why free sugars consumption

should be below 15 kg per person per year in industrialised countries: the dental evidence. *Br Dent J,* 1991;171:63-5.

158. Mondini L, Monteiro CA. Mudanças no padrão de alimentação. *In:* Monteiro CA, editor. *Velhos e novos males da saúde no Brasil: a evolução do país e suas doenças.* São Paulo, HUCITEC/NUPENS/USP; 2000.
159. World Health Organization. *Diet, nutrition, and the prevention of chronic diseases.* Geneva: WHO; 1990. Technical Report Series 797.
160. Moura MS, Santos-Pinto LAM, Giro EMA, Cordeiro RCL. Cárie dentária relacionada ao nível socioeconômico em escolares de Araraquara. *Rev Odontol Univ São Paulo,*1996;25(1):97-107.
161. Morais ND, Lenza MA, Freire MCM. Prevalência de cárie em escolares de 6 a 12 anos da rede pública de ensino do município de Dom Aquino-MT. *Rev Bras Odontol Saúde Coletiva,* 2000, jul/dez; 1(2): 45-9.
162. Pattussi MP. As desigualdades na distribuição da cárie dentária em escolares de 12 anos residentes em diferentes regiões socioeconômicas do Distrito Federal, Brasil – 1997. *Rev Bras Odontol Saúde Coletiva* 2000, jan/jun; 1(1):19-28.
163. Maltz M, Silva BB. Relação entre cárie, gengivite e fluorose e nível socioeconômico em escolares. *Rev Saúde Pública,* 2001;35(2):170-6.
164. Gillespie S. Policy priorities: themes and action. *In:* Flores R, Gillespie S. *Health and nutrition: emerging and reemerging issues in developing countries.* Washington: International Food Policy Research Institute/2020 Vision; Feb 2001. Focus 5. Brief 11.
165. Cannon GJ. In: Flores R, Gillespie S. *Health and nutrition: emerging and reemerging issues in developing countries.* Washington: International Food Policy Research Institute/2020 Vision; Feb 2001. Focus 5. Brief 8.
166. Croucher R. General dental practice, health education, and health promotion: a critical reappraisal. *In:* Schou L, Blinkhorn AS, editors. *Oral Health Promotion.* Oxford: Oxford Medical Publications; 1993. p.153-68.
167. World Health Organization. Otawa Charter for health promotion. *Health Promotion* 1987;1(44): iii-v.
168. Sheiham A. Integrating dental care with general health care. *World Health,* 1988, Oct; 28-9.
169. Sheiham A. The role of the dental team in promoting dental health and general health through oral health. *Int Dent J,* 1992;42:223-8.
170. Prefeitura de Curitiba. *Abastecimento.* Disponível em: URL:http://www.curitiba.pr.gov.br/pmc/editorias/asp [2002 Jun 17]
171. Anônimo. Superando expectativas. *Prom Saúde,* 2001; 2(5): 29-30.
172. Sanderson ME. *Towards a sugar health policy* [dissertation]. Cranfield Institute of Technology; 1984.
173. Sanderson ME. O caminho do futuro: a força motriz da política do açúcar. In: ABOPREV. *Prática odontológica centrada em prevenção: aspectos básicos.* São Paulo, ABOPREV; 1991. Biblioteca Científica, Fascículo 2 - Açúcares: debate atual e ação futura.
174. Cannon GJ. *Food and health: the experts agree.* London: Consumers' Association; 1992.
175. NFA/WCRF. 5+Everyday. London: NFA/WCRF; 1997.
176. Freire MCM. *An analysis of recommendations on sugar consumption from national dietary guidelines* [dissertation]. London: Department of Community Dental Health - University College London; 1991.
177. Freire MCM, Cannon GJ, Sheiham A. Análise das recomendações internacionais sobre o consumo de açúcares publicadas entre 1961 e 1991. *Rev Saúde Públ,* 1994;28:228-37.
178. Department of Health. *Dietary reference values for food energy and nutrients for the United Kingdom.* Report of the panel on dietary reference values of the Committee on Medical Aspects of Food Policy. London: HMSO; 1991. Report on Health and Social Subjects No. 41.
179. Bengoa JM, Torun B, Behar M, Scrimshaw NS. Nutritional goals for health in Latin America. *Food Nutr Bull,* 1989;11(1):4-20.
180. Vannucchi H, Menezes EW, Campana AO, Lajolo FM. *Aplicações das recomendações nutricionais adaptadas à população brasileira.* Ribeirão Preto: SBAN; 1990. Cadernos de Nutrição, 2.

Chapter 8

Effective Caries Prevention with Fluoride

Valéria Coelho Catão Marinho

Introduction

Fluoride therapy has been the centerpiece of caries-preventive strategies since the introduction of water fluoridation schemes over five decades ago. However, while everyone agrees that the methods used in the prevention and treatment of dental caries should be effective, there is a surprising difference of opinions as to what is the best means of achieving caries prevention and how to obtain the best results through the appropriate use of fluorides.

Differences of opinion and practice exist as shown by the variations in the patterns of fluoride use from country to country and within a country, and from practice to practice. These variations exist for all types of fluoride-based measures. For example, strong views are held both for and against water fluoridation, which have promoted or prevented its adoption in many countries. Dentifrices containing fluoride are the most widespread form of fluoride usage nowadays, but as the prevalence of caries has decreased, and concern has been expressed that fluorosis has increased, the early use of fluoride toothpaste by children has been under scrutiny in various settings. This has raised the question of what should the optimum level of fluoride be in toothpastes used by children. A variety of topical fluoride treatments in the form of gels, varnishes and rinses are used in public health programmes, clinical practice, or individually at home, and some of these may be used at the same time in different combinations, in communities where the water is fluoridated and where toothpaste use is ubiquitous.

A number of factors may explain the variations in the patterns of fluoride use. Some factors relate to differences in the needs of the recipients of care such as their caries levels. Other factors reflect differences in the availability of resources or in the way oral health care is financed and provided and differences in influences from manufacturers, organizations and others.

One of the most important, if not the most important determinant of variations in preventive practice in relation to fluoride, is the uncertainty that exists among those who make decisions in oral health care about the effectiveness and safety of the main forms of fluoride interventions currently in use for the control of dental caries in children. The evidence available on the effectiveness and safety of fluorides is the focus of this chapter. First, the rationale and methods that have been used to arrive at the summaries and conclusions on the topic will be outlined. Then, the latest evidence available on the effectiveness and safety of the various forms of fluoride will be presented.

Scientific basis for evaluating the effectiveness of preventive interventions

The basis for prioritizing one of a number of alternative forms of care can sometimes be based on no more than a subjective impression that it is superior. But it is essential that this is confirmed or refuted by the results of properly conducted studies, because obtaining the best scientific evidence to help guide treatment decisions should be a fundamental aim of those engaged in health care research and practice. Unless formal evaluations are done, effective forms of care will not be recognized as such, and brought into use as promptly as possible, ineffective or harmful forms of care will not be detected and avoided efficiently, and the uncertainty about the effects, both beneficial and adverse, of many other forms of care will not be made explicit (Chalmers et al, 1997).

There are current debates about the appropriate use of various forms of fluoride. The questions being asked relate to their actual effectiveness and the potential risks (mainly in terms of fluorosis) that may be expected from the various fluoride based caries preventive measures in an era of decreased caries prevalence and widespread availability of fluoride from multiple sources. The persistence of this debate and the variations in the patterns of fluoride use suggest the need to focus on the scientific basis for the appropriate use of fluorides.

A large number of formal studies attempts to address uncertainties about the effects of the many forms of fluoride interventions. This is perhaps unsurprising, as fluoride has been the object of basic and clinical research for over 50 years. A simple search of MEDLINE (an electronic bibliographic database which covers all areas of medicine, nursery, dentistry, and basic clinical sciences) for the text words 'fluoride' or 'fluoride AND caries', covering the years 1965 to 1999, can be used to provide a picture of the considerable amount of any type of research published on the topic in the last four decades (Fig.8.1).

Separate free text searches have been carried out to call attention to the fact that not all the research on the subject is related to caries alone (however, there have probably been more reports in the dental literature on the caries-inhibitory property of fluoride than on any other aspect of dentistry). Combining each of the subject search terms above with specific methodological filters provide an indication of the amount of research addressing questions related to the effects of fluoride, and recommendations for the appropriate use of fluorides (the epidemiology of different 'levels' of research about effectiveness on fluoride).

Not all of these studies, however, provide reliable information. If judgements about the effectiveness (and safety) of health care interventions based on formal studies are to be valid, careful consideration must be given to the strengths and weaknesses of the methods used by the investigators. In this way a rational basis can be established for selecting those studies that are most likely to provide useful and valid evidence.

Box 8.1 Number and types of publications about fluorides and fluorides and caries, 1966-1999 (results from a MEDLINE search using the text words 'fluoride', and 'fluoride and caries').

The Epidemiology of Different "Levels" of Research on Fluor (Medline Search)

Fluor* = 26.526	Fluor* + Carie* = 6.799
• Review articles	• Review articles
– Sistematic/meta-analyses = 22	– Sistematic/meta-analyses = 19
– Reviews = 534	– Reviews = 244
• Guidelines	• Guidelines
– Guidelines = 30	– Guidelines = 11
– Consensus/guidelines/ recommend* = 514	– Consensus/guidelines/ recommend* = 228
• Clinical trials = 1.198	• Clinical trials = 602
• Other integrative and primary studies	• Other integrative and primary studies

The usefulness and validity of the best evidence about effectiveness: levels ofevidence and quality of randomized controlled trials (RCTs) and systematic reviews

When considering the usefulness of the available evidence from research about effectiveness it is essential to highlight the fact that some types of evidence are more reliable than other types, i.e. the strength of inference one can draw from a particular piece of research depends on the method used to conduct it. The following table provides a guide to the different levels of evidence available and their relative strengths, where type I evidence is the strongest and type V is the weakest (Table 8.1).

This hierarchy of strength of evidence reflects the degree to which different methods of assessing the effects of health care interventions on important outcomes are susceptible to bias (or systematic errors) that may render their results less reliable for making inferences. The levels of research evidence about effectiveness range from simple descriptive studies (e.g. case reports, cross-sectional and ecological studies) through observational studies of indi-

Table 8.1 The five types and strengths of research evidence about effectiveness (Gray, 1997).

Type	Strength of Evidence
I	Strong evidence from at least one systematic review of multiple well designed RCTs
II	Strong evidence from at least one well designed RCT of appropriate size
III	Evidence from controlled trials without randomization, or from observational studies (cohort, single group pre-post, time series or case-control studies)
IV	Evidence from well designed non-experimental studies from more than one center or research groups
V	Evidence from reports of expert committees based on the sources of evidence cited, descriptive studies (cross-sectional, ecological studies, case series) or opinions of respected authorities based on clinical evidence

vidual based associations (e.g. case-control and cohort studies), to formal experiments (e.g. randomized controlled trials) and systematic reviews:

Case Report and Case Series

Analysis of one case or of a series of people with the condition/exposure. There is no comparison group in case series, or in single case reports. (Unless the effects of care are dramatic and unambiguous (and this is rare), these studies can only provide very weak evidence, as they are subject to a variety of biases that may be sufficiently large either to mask real differences in effect, or to suggest that differences exist when, in fact, they do not.)

Cross Sectional Study

A study design that involves surveying a population about an exposure, or condition, or both, at one point in time, to investigate the prevalence of a condition/exposure. There is no comparison group in a cross sectional study. (These studies are often difficult to interpret, as it is not possible to assess whether the outcome followed the exposure or the exposure resulted from the outcome.)

Ecological Study

A study design that looks at disease occurrence, especially with regard to an environmental exposure determined by geography, where the average exposure of the population is plotted against the rate of the outcome for that population to investigate any possible association between the two. (These studies are considered to provide weak evidence about effectiveness because of concern about compatibility of information from different areas, data is often unavailable on many risk factors, and because of uncertainties in extrapolating results of analyses at population level to the individual.)

Case Control Study

A study design that examines a group of people who have experienced a particular event/outcome (usually an adverse event) and a group of people who have not experienced the same event, and looks at how exposure to suspect agents differed between the two groups. (This type of study is most useful for trying to ascertain the cause of rare events. Conclusions about causes and effects are often insecure though, as no amount of matching using information about known confounding factors can ever eliminate the effect of unknown confounding factors).

Cohort Study

A study that examines a cohort (group of people) separated into one of two or more study groups depending on whether they have or have not been exposed to the agent under investigation. The selected groups are followed-up for a period of time in order to measure the frequency of occurrence of the outcomes of interest in those exposed compared to those not exposed to try to ascertain whether exposure is likely to cause the events. (This type of study is unbiased in terms of disease development, time-order relationships are known, but potential weaknesses include loss to follow-up, changes in subjects characteristics, and surveillance bias where one group is observed in more detail than the other.)

Historical Co7ntrol Study

This is one approach to the selection of controls that involves making comparisons between people who have received a recently introduced form of care with similar people who received a different form of care in the past. (This type of study is most useful as 'screening tests' for promising new forms of care, because without concurrent comparisons there is no way of knowing which of the studies using historical controls provide reliable data about the effects of care, and which do not. It can sometimes be misleading because even when outcome following current treatment appears to differ substantially from outcome following earlier forms of care, this may be a reflection of changes in undocumented factors that have modified the outcome over time.)

Randomized Control trial (RCT)

An experimental study in which people are assigned randomly to two or more groups, at least one (experimental group) receiving an intervention that is being tested and another (control group) receiving an alternative treatment or placebo. The outcomes of interest are compared at the end of a given follow-up time. Any observed differences in outcome should reflect differences in the effectiveness of the interventions compared.

Systematic review and meta-analysis

A piece of research carried out to identify, appraise, and summarize the results and implications of otherwise unmanageable quantities of research addressing a defined question in order to provide an unbiased summary of the evidence by following an objective and methodologically rigorous approach. It can, but need not, involve meta-analysis. Meta-analysis is a statistical technique that combines the results of several studies in a single weighted estimate, in which more weight is given to results of studies with more events/larger samples.

While variations of the hierarchy of evidence based on the study designs described above are still being proposed and employed by health scientists (Woolf et al, 1990; Guyatt et al, 1995), those who have proposed the variations seem to agree that with regard to primary study methodology randomized trials should be considered the most reliable method of assembling comparison groups on which to base causal inferences about the effects of care (Kleijnen et al, 1997). It is important to note that ranked above experimental studies of adequate size using proper randomization are scientific quantitative summaries of such studies, namely, systematic reviews using meta-analysis of multiple well-designed RCTs.

A consensus is growing that the most valid answers to important health care questions will come from such reviews based on rigorous research methods, and the most obvious manifestation of this trend is the international Cochrane Collaboration, a worldwide attempt to prepare and disseminate systematic reviews of randomized controlled trials of the effects of health care interventions (Chalmers et al, 1992; Clarke and Langhorne, 2001).

Cochrane reviews

These are systematic reviews of randomized controlled trials maintained by contributors to the Cochrane Collaboration. Published in an electronic form the reviews have advantages over more traditional methods: they are updated as new evidence emerges and mistakes can be corrected in response to comments and criticisms. The review thereby continues to be the best single place where a distillation of the latest evidence is easily accessible. The full text of each of the reviews is available in the Cochrane Database of Systematic Reviews (CDSR) in The Cochrane Library.

Thus, the strongest scientific evidence about effectiveness will come from quantitative study designs that are likely to provide the best means of minimizing or avoiding systematic errors (or bias), and also have a number (and variety) of observations from randomized evidence which is large enough to control for random errors (or chance effects). This is because in most circumstances, the effect of an intervention will not be very large. So a large amount of randomized evidence is needed to detect or refute reliably such moderate, but potentially worthwhile effects (Clarke and Stewart, 1994). Evidence from non randomized controlled trials, unduly small randomized trials, or unduly small systematic reviews of (smaller) randomized trials are all inferior as sources of evidence about effectiveness. They cannot discriminate reliably between moderate and negligible differences in outcome; and such non-randomized or small-scale inconclusive evidence may yield wrong conclusions (Peto, 1987; Collins et al, 1997).

However, lack of money, resources and time may limit the size of an experimental study, and consequently evidence from large randomized trials or from conclusive systematic reviews with meta-analysis of such trials will be unavailable for most health care interventions, before they become widely accepted or rejected prematurely. Therefore, systematic reviews that are based on meta-analysis of existing randomized trials are the most appropriate research methodology for providing the best available evidence about effectiveness (Chalmers et al, 1992; Chalmers and Lau, 1993; Egger et al, 1997).

* Quality of a study is defined as the confidence that its design anda analysis has minimized or avoided bias.

The caveat is that all the research must be of high quality[1]. And study quality will not only depend on the strength of the design used, which very much relates to the question the study is trying to answer, but also on how well the study has been carried out and reported.

The critical appraisal of the quality of RCTs and systematic reviews

The factors that are important when conducting and reporting clinical trials and reviews are also important when critically appraising their quality. A few basic criteria for quality assessment should be followed. And even though it might not be possible to answer all the questions on the basis of the published reports alone, they will be of help in the cautious interpretation of the results of these reports.

The most widely used self-directed critical appraisal criteria have been generated by the Evidence-Based Medicine Working Group at McMaster University: the so-called "JAMA (Journal of the American Medical Association) series" of user's guides to the health care literature (Guyatt and Rennie, 1993). Two sets of critical appraisal questions adapted from these series, for evaluating the validity of original articles (controlled trials) and review articles (systematic reviews/ meta-analises) on the effects of therapy or prevention are presented in Tables 8.2 and 8.3 (Guyatt et al, 1993; Guyatt et al, 1994; Oxman et al, 1994).

They focus on flaws in study design and implementation that are most likely to weaken the strength of inference in ways that may seriously distort decisions based on them.

Table 8.2 Basic critical appraisal questions for evaluating the quality of a controlled trial (Guyatt et al, 1993; Guyatt et al, 1994). Each can be answered "Yes, Can't tell, No".

- Are the results of the study valid, i.e. how close to the truth are they?
- Was the assignment of people to treatment randomized? And was randomization concealed?
- Were all those who entered the trial properly accounted for at its conclusion and analyzed in the groups to which they were randomized?
- Were participants, outcome assessors and care givers 'blind' to treatment?
- Aside from the experimental intervention, were the groups treated equally?
- Were the groups similar at the start of the trial?

Table 8.3 Basic critical appraisal questions for evaluating the quality of a review article (Oxman et al, 1994). Each can be answered "Yes, Can't tell, No".

- Are the results of the study valid, i.e. how close to the truth are they?
- Were the objectives clearly stated?
- Were the inclusion criteria for studies selection explicit and appropriate?
- Were the methods used to find studies stated and comprehensive?
- Was the methodological quality of included studies assessed using appropriate criteria?
- Were selection and assessments of studies reproducible?
- Were any differences in study results adequately explained?
- Were results combined appropriately relative to the question addressed?

In RCTs, bias can be reflected in systematic differences between the comparison groups in the participants' characteristics (selection bias), in the care provided apart from the intervention being evaluated (performance bias), in outcome assessment (detection bias), and in the occurrence and handling of withdrawals from the trial (exclusion or attrition bias) (Altman, 1991). Thus, RCTs should be routinely scrutinized for such methodological flaws, which may threaten the validity of their findings.

In systematic reviews, bias can be reflected in the methods used to identify studies for inclusion in the review (publication bias, language bias, database bias, citation bias), to determine eligibility of the studies for inclusion (inclusion criteria bias) and to assess their quality (quality scoring bias), and in the methods used to extract accurate relevant data (extractor bias, outcome reporting bias, data provision bias). Thus, systematic reviews of RCTs also need to be carefully appraised, since they are susceptible to potential sources of bias inherent to retrospective studies.

Studies have shown that Cochrane reviews are, on average, more systematic and less biased than other systematic reviews published in high-profile paper journals (Egger et al 1997; Jadad et al, 1998; Jadad et al, 2000; Shea et al, 2001). However, they can also contain some problems in how they were conducted and reported (Olsen et al, 2001). Therefore, regardless of the source of publication, all systematic reviews (like all types of research evidence) require critical appraisal to determine their validity and to establish whether and how they will be used in practice (Hunt and McKibbon, 1997).

The precision of the findings of RCTs and systematic reviews

Even after successful control of biases that may distort comparisons of alternative forms of care in RCTs and systematic reviews, the results of such comparisons may still be misleading because of random errors. Random errors will be reduced as samples yielding larger numbers of the outcomes of interest are studied; i.e. in large trials and in systematic reviews incorporating all the available data from broadly similar trials. Estimating the range within which the true differential effect of alternative forms of care is likely to lie, by calculating a confidence interval for the statistical estimate of the differences in outcome(s), provides further protection against being misled by random errors, in both RCTs and systematic reviews of RCTs. The breadth of the confidence interval denotes the precision of the difference in effect (the level of uncertainty around the finding).

Confidence interval (CI)

An interval within which the population parameter (the 'true' effect) is expected to lie with a given degree of certainty (usually 95%). The 95% confidence interval (or confidence limit) would include 95% of results from studies of the same size and design in the same population. (The practical advantage of a confidence interval, rather than a P value is that it presents the range of likely effects).

Nevertheless, systematic deviations from the truth can be considered worse than errors that occur by chance alone in systematic reviews. Because if the review has been carefully conducted and quantitative results are derived using meta-analysis of all available relevant evidence, the confidence intervals around the results will indicate the 'precision', or the likelihood of such chance effects (Oxman, 1994). As more participants will be included in a systematic review than in any individual study that contributes to it, chance effects will tend to be minimized in meta-analyses of published and unpublished studies.

On the other hand, although otherwise well-designed randomized trials may offer protection against the possibility of being misled by bias, too often they provide little protection by being misled by the play of chance (random errors) due to small sample sizes (or low power to detect an effect if it exists). One consequence of this problem is that forms of care that do have differential effects of practical importance are deemed to be equivalent. This adds to the importance of compiling similar studies together in systematic reviews.

The balance of beneficial and harmful effects in studies designed to assess effectiveness

Finding high quality evidence on negative or adverse effects of treatment is even more difficult. Although RCTs and systematic reviews are powerful research methods to assess beneficial effects of health care interventions, many trials are not sufficiently large or long term to capture rarer effects or effects that occur later, after a few years, and many do not adequately report adverse effects. If the adverse effect is mild, for example, mild fluorosis, this may not be crucial, but if the effect is fluorosis of aesthetic concern, symptoms of acute fluoride toxicity, or bone fracture, this can be very important. Therefore, weaker levels of evidence; i.e. study designs such as observational studies designed to assess safety often need to be considered in order to complement RCTs designed to assess effectiveness, especially when the potential harm is serious. It is generally recognized however that the reporting of potential harmful effects in effectiveness evaluations, especially in systematic reviews, requires further work.

Moreover, in order to get the reporting of effectiveness right for any particular intervention it is important to make a clear distinction between 'lack of benefit' (when there is good evidence that the treatment is unlikely to be beneficial) and 'lack of evidence of benefit' (there is no good evidence that a treatment does more good than harm).

The applicability of results from research about effectiveness

Even if one is reasonably certain that bias and chance effects have been adequately controlled in a particular study or in a systematic review of similar studies, questions may remain about the extent to which this research evidence constitutes a valid basis for guiding practice.

Sometimes, the limited applicability of the findings may be relatively clear (the 'external validity' of the findings may be compromised either because there are crucial differences between participants in formal investigations and people receiving the intervention in other contexts, or because the nature of the health care intervention provided within formal comparisons and that provided in usual practice differ). More often, however, it will not be possible to conclude with confidence that the evidence is not applicable in practice, i.e. there will not be a compelling reason why the evidence should not be applicable, especially if the evidence is from a systematic review where results are consistent across many high quality studies (Guyatt et al 1994).

In addition, any real differences in the effects of care that exist between participants in controlled trials/reviews of trials and similar people seen in the context of day to day practice are more likely to be differences in the magnitude of effects than differences in the direction of effects (Yusuf et al, 1991). Judgements to guide practice must then be made more in terms of whether the magnitude of the differential effect is sufficient to warrant modification of usual practice.

Therefore, having identified the evidence that may be both useful and valid will not automatically dictate what to do by providing gold standard answers, but

cepted that any pre-eruptive benefit from ingestion of fluoride during tooth development is relatively unimportant. Thus, they have a poor risk benefit trade-off. In addition, because tablets and supplements carry considerable difficulties for regular and appropriate use, it is becoming increasingly more difficult to justify their adoption as a public health measure.

The identification of systematic reviews on the effects of fluoride

The evidence on the effects of water fluoridation and topical fluorides (toothpastes, mouthrinses, gels and varnishes) was located by database searches specifically performed to collect information on existing and ongoing systematic reviews/meta-analyses. The Cochrane Library databases – the Cochrane Database of Systematic Reviews (CDSR) and the Database of Abstracts of Reviews of Effects (DARE) – and MEDLINE were searched.

MEDLINE remains the standard bibliographic database for biomedical information, and can be easily searched on-line, using Pub Med (http://www.ncbi.nlm.nih.gov/PubMed/), the US National Library of Medicine's electronic index of nearly 4500 journals from over 70 countries. Because many published review articles are unsystematic, methodological 'filters' most likely to retrieve systematic reviews/meta-analyses were used for the MEDLINE search. Methodological terms were not needed to search the relevant specialized databases in the Cochrane Library. Many if not the majority of, existing systematic reviews in the dental field (including ongoing reviews in the form of protocols) can be found directly in the CDSR and in the DARE databases in The Cochrane Library. This electronic source of reliable and continuously updated information includes specialized databases with all full text reviews prepared by the Cochrane Collaboration (in the CDSR) and with critical assessments and structured abstracts of systematic reviews published elsewhere and critically appraised by the NHS Centre for Reviews and Dissemination at the University of York, UK (in the DARE).

Since 2000, Cochrane reviews are indexed in MEDLINE, and this has made it easier to identify these maintained systematic reviews and to keep track of them (Clarke and Oxman 1999; Kotzin 2002). Structured abstracts that convey essential information in a standardized format are included in the MEDLINE file without modification. The abstracts of all Cochrane reviews (over 1500 reviews as of October 2002) are also available on the Web via the publisher's site (http://www.update-software.com/Cochrane/abstract.htm).

Fourteen relevant reviews were identified in the search and assessed further. Two early studies that have used the meta-analytical approach have been published nearly two decades ago. One is a review of US fluoride mouthrinses studies in fluoride deficient communities (Stamm et al, 1984) and the other is a study by Clark et al (1985) on the comparative effectiveness of acidulated phosphate fluoride (APF) gels and solutions and fluoride varnishes. However, these reviews are not considered further due to the several methodological (and applicability) limitations that characterize these early attempts to quantitative synthesis in the dental field.

A few meta-analyses on the effects of topical fluoride therapy were published in the 1990s. Two of them address the comparative efficacy of two commercially available active forms of fluoride in toothpaste (Johnson 1993; Stamm 1995). Another is a meta-analysis on the effectiveness of one commercially available fluoride varnish system, Duraphat (Helfenstein and Steiner, 1994; 1994a) and the other is a meta-analysis on the effectiveness of fluoride gels (van Rijkom, 1998). A common

Table 8.4 The main features and the results of the reviews/meta-analyses published in the 1990's on the effects of topical fluoride interventions.

Study	Focus	Inclusion criteria	Search/Selection/ Quality assesment/ Data extraction	Statistical analysis/ Investigation of heterogeneity/Findings
Van Rijkom,[25] 1998	An investigation on the caries-inhibiting effect of fluoride gel treatment in children and on factors potentially modifying this effect.	Randomized studies on fluoride gels (versus placebo or no treatment), applied to permanent teeth of children aged six to 15 years, in the general population. Outcome measure: caries increment	MEDLINE (1965 to 1995) was searched for English and German language papers. Studies selected independently by 2 examiners, but no report on method for assessing validity, or on how many performed the validity assessment and data extraction.	17 studies analyzed (8263 participants) – caries reduction was 22% (95% CI: 18, 25%) favoring fluoride gels. Differences in caries increment expressed as Prevented Fractions (PF). Model used for MA not reported. Multiple regression analysis showed no significant influence on the PF for the variables "baseline caries prevalence", "general fluoride regimen", "application method" (tray/brush), and "application frequency".
Stamm,[24] 1995	Comparative efficacy of two formulations of fluoride dentifrices: sodium fluoride (NAF) and sodium monofluorophosphate (SMFP).	Not specified in terms of participants/outcomes. Study design/ interventions: RCTs reporting direct comparison of the two agents, and "appropriateness" of the test agents.	Not reported.	12 studies analyzed (14,257 participants) – difference in efficacy was 7% favoring NaF toothpaste. Differences in caries increment expressed as standardized mean differences in D(M)FS. Fixed effects model used for conventional and cumulative meta-analysis. Heterogeneity not investigated.
Johnson,[22] 1993	Comparative efficacy of two formulations of fluoride dentifrices: sodium fluoride (NAF) and sodium mono-fluorophosphate (SMFP).	Not specified in terms of participants. Study design/interventions: RCTs reporting direct comparison of the two agents, and Anticalculus studies, and Dual-active studies. Outcome: caries increment	Published studies searched. ("Design" rating used but in another publication). Study identification and selection processes not reported. Quality assessment and data extraction methods not reported.	9 head -to- head studies (over 7000 participants) – overall weighted mean difference of 0..28 (95% CI: 0.10, 0.46) favoring NaF toothpaste (representing a 6.4% reduction in the rate of caries development). Differences in caries increment expressed as weighted absolute mean differences in D(M)FS. Fixed effects and random effects model used for meta-analyses performed. Tests of heterogeneity performed. Sensitiv ity analyses performed
Helfenstein e Steiner,[23] 1994[23]	An investigation on the caries preventive effects of	Specified in terms of participants (children aged 6-15), intervention (Duraphat), outcome measures (caries increment) and study design (not restricted to RCTs).	Searched Index to Dental Literature 1985-91 and references from review articles. Study identification and study selection processes not described. Judgments on validity and data extraction method not reported.	9 studies analyzed (1851 participants) – caries reduction was 38% (95% CI: 19%, 57%) favoring fluoride varnish. Differences in caries increment expressed as weighted mean differences in D(M)FS. Random effects model used for meta-analysis. Test of heterogeneity significant. Influence of study duration observed (effect decreased with time). Sensitivity analyses performed (not specified a priori): fixed effects model used.

feature present in the first three studies is a greater focus on the statistical aspects of the investigation, rather than on the clinical and public health implications. Table 8.4 shows the main features and the results of the four reviews.

Not until 2000 was a systematic review published on the body of evidence available on the efficacy and safety of water fluoridation (McDonagh et al, 2000). Apart from being available in the form of a journal article, the full version of the published report is also available on the Web (http://www.york.ac.uk/inst/crd/fluorid.htm). The main features of the review, results and conclusions, are presented in the next section.

In July 2003, 7 Cochrane systematic reviews (Table 8.5) were available on the effects topical fluoride interventions, four of which as complete systematic reviews and three as protocols of on-going reviews (The Cochrane Library Issue 2, 2003). The Cochrane reviews on fluoride toothpastes, mouthrinses, gels, and varnishes are also considered in detail in the next sections (Marinho et al, 2002; Marinho et al, 2002a; Marinho et al, 2003, Marinho et al, 2003a). Abstracts of these reviews are available on the Cochrane Oral Health Group web site (http://www.cochrane-oral.man.ac.uk)

It is important to point out that the full text of these and all other Cochrane reviews are available free of charge to an increasing number of countries where access to The Cochrane Library on-line is provided to everybody (national provision): Australia, England, Wales, Ireland, Finland and Norway. In Brazil, BIREME provides online access to The Cochrane Library through the BIREME interface (in English, Spanish or Portuguese) free of charge (http://www.bireme.br). Free access will soon be extended to all countries in Latin and Central America and the Caribbean. In South Africa, free access to The Cochrane Library is available for registered members of SA HealthInfo. And through a partnership led by WHO, free access to The Cochrane Library is also provided at least for 100 low-income countries.

Evidence on the effects of fluoride-based treatments for the prevention of dental caries in children

6.1 Water fluoridation

The evidence reviewed

NHS CRD. A systematic review of public water fluoridation. York: NHS Centre for Reviews and Dissemination. University of York, 2000. (http://www.york.ac.uk/inst/crd/fluorid.htm)

McDonagh MS, Whiting PF, Wilson PM, Sutton AJ, Chestnutt I, Cooper J, et al. Systematic review of water fluoridation. BMJ 2000; 321: 855-859. (http://bmj.com/cgi/content/full/321/7265/855)

Objectives of the review

The aim of this report was to assess the evidence on the positive and negative effects of population wide drinking water fluoridation strategies to prevent caries. To achieve this aim five objectives were identified:

1. What are the effects of fluoridation of drinking water supplies on the incidence of caries?
2. If water fluoridation is shown to have beneficial effects, what is the effect over and above that offered by the use of alternative interventions and strategies?
3. Does water fluoridation result in a reduction of caries across social groups and between geographical locations, bringing equity?

4. Does water fluoridation have negative effects?

5. Are there differences in the effects of natural and artificial water fluoridation?

Interventions included in the review

Water fluoridation.

Participants included in the review

Populations receiving fluoridated water (largely children).

Outcomes assessed in the review

Two main outcomes were considered for assessment of efficacy, decayed, (missing) and filled primary and permanent teeth at baseline and at the final examination, and the proportion of children without caries. Several indices were used to classify enamel opacities, including fluorosis. Dental fluorosis was defined as any score other than normal in each index used. A second method to account for fluorosis of aesthetic concern was selected, but only data from studies reporting on chosen indices could be used.

Study designs included in the review

Studies were classified into the levels of evidence. Evidence rated below a level of moderate quality/moderate risk of bias (level B, equivalent to type III in table 10.1) was not considered in the evaluation of efficacy. In the assessment of safety, all levels of evidence were considered.

Table 8.5 The 7 Cochrane reviews available on the effects of topical fluoride (The Cochrane Library Issue 1, 2003).

Reviews

- Fluoride toothpastes for preventing dental caries in children and adolescents
- Fluoride gels for preventing dental caries in children and adolescents
- Fluoride varnishes for preventing dental caries in children and adolescents
- Fluoride rinses for preventing dental caries in children and adolescents

Protocols

- Topical fluoride (toothpastes, mouthrinses, gels or varnishes) for preventing dental caries in children and adolescents
- One topical fluoride (varnishes, or gels, or rinses, or toothpastes) versus another for preventing dental caries in children and adolescents
- Combinations of topical fluorides (varnishes, gels, rinses, toothpastes) versus one topical fluoride for preventing dental caries in children and adolescents

Sources searched

Searches of 25 electronic databases, of bibliographies of included studies, and the World Wide Web were undertaken. Published and unpublished studies in any language were sought.

Data collection process (study selection, quality assessment, data extraction)

Inclusion decisions, quality assessment and data extraction were duplicated by two reviewers, and consensus achieved by discussion or a third party.

Data analysis process (measures of treatment effect, meta-analysis, examination of sources of differences between studies)

The primary measure of effect was the difference of the change in caries prevalence from baseline to the final examination in the fluoridated area compared with the control area in children of the same age. Random effects meta-analyses were performed where data could be pooled. Potential sources of heterogeneity were examined in random effects meta-regression analyses (effect of baseline levels of caries, age, study duration, validity scores, and others). Multi-level regression analysis was used to combine studies and investigate the association of water fluoride concentration with the prevalence of fluorosis.

Results of the review

There were 214 studies included; none was of evidence level A (high quality, bias unlikely). The study designs used included 102 cross sectional studies, 47 ecological studies, 45 controlled before-after studies, seven case control studies, and 13 cohort studies.

Objective 1

The best available evidence (level B – 23 before-after studies and three cohort studies) from studies on the initiation and discontinuation of water fluoridation suggests that fluoridation does reduce caries prevalence, both as measured by the proportion of children who are caries-free and by the mean dmft/DMFT score. The degree to which caries is reduced, however, is not clear from the data available: The range (median) of the mean difference in the proportion of children without caries was – 5.0% to 64% (14.6%), the range (median) of mean change in decayed, missing and filled primary/permanent teeth was 0.5 to 4.4 (2.25) teeth. There was significant heterogeneity among the included studies. Meta-regression showed that the proportion of children without caries at baseline, the setting, and the validity score show a significant association with the difference in risk in the proportion of children without caries. Baseline decayed, missing, and filled primary/permanent teeth, age, setting, and duration of study show a significant association with the mean difference in decayed, missing, and filled primary/permanent teeth.

Objective 2

An effect of water fluoridation was still evident in studies completed after 1974 in spite of the assumed exposure to fluoride from other sources by the populations studied. The meta-regression conducted for Objective 1 confirmed this finding. The studies included for Objective 2 were also of moderate quality (level B), but of limited quantity. Thus, the power to detect a difference may have been limited. In addition, using the date of publication may not have been sufficiently sensitive to identify any change.

Objective 3

The available evidence on social class effects of water fluoridation in reducing caries appears to suggest a benefit in reducing the differences in severity of tooth decay (as measured by dmft/DMFT) between classes among five and 12 year-old children. No effect on the overall measure of proportion of caries-free children was detected. However, the quality of the evidence is low (level C), and based on a small number of studies. Thus, the association between water fluoridation, caries and social class needs further clarification.

Objective 4

The possible negative effects of water fluoridation were examined as broadly as possible. The effects on dental fluorosis are the clearest. There is a dose-response relationship between water fluoride level and the prevalence of fluorosis (shown in the meta-regression analysis). Fluorosis appears to occur frequently at fluoride levels typically used in artificial fluoridation schemes. The proportion of fluorosis that is aesthetically concerning is lower: the pooled estimate of the prevalence of fluorosis at a water fluoride concentration of 1.0 ppm was 48% (95% confidence interval 40% to 57%) and for fluorosis of aesthetic concern 12.5% (95% confidence interval 7.0% to 21.5%). There was, however, considerable heterogeneity between results of individual studies. Although 88 studies of fluorosis were included, they were of low quality (level C – most of the studies were cross sectional, only four were controlled before-after studies). In addition, observer bias may be of importance in studies assessing fluorosis, but efforts to reduce this potential bias or to control for potential confounding factors were uncommon in the included studies.

The best available evidence on the association of water fluoridation and bone fractures show no definite patterns of association. Similarly, the best available evidence on the association of water fluoridation and cancers show no clear association. The miscellaneous other adverse effects studied did not provide enough good quality evidence on any particular outcome to reach conclusions. The outcomes related to infant mortality, congenital defects and IQ indicate a need for further high quality research, using appropriate analytical methods to control for confounding factors. While fluorosis can occur within a few years of exposure during tooth development, other potential adverse effects may require long-term exposure to occur. It is possible that this long-term exposure has not been captured by these studies.

Objective 5

The evidence on natural versus artificial fluoride sources was extremely limited, and direct comparisons were not possible for most outcomes. While no major differences were apparent in this review, the evidence is not adequate to reach a conclusion regarding this objective.

Reviewers' conclusions

This review presents a summary of the best available and most reliable evidence on the safety and efficacy of water fluoridation. Given the level of interest surrounding the issue of public water fluoridation, it is surprising to find that little high quality research has been undertaken. As such, this review should provide both researchers and commissioners of research with an overview of the methodological limitations of previous research conducted in this area. The evidence of a benefit of a reduction in caries should be considered together with the increased prevalence of dental fluorosis. The research evidence is of insufficient quality to allow confident statements about other potential harms or whether there is an impact on social inequalities. (No clear evidence of other potential negative effects was found; thus, a message of no evidence of harm is not to be conveyed). Thus, caution against overinterpretation of the results

Medicine Working Group. *JAMA*, 1994; 272(17):1367-1371.
13. Hunt DL, McKibbon KA. Locating and appraising systematic reviews. *Ann Intern Med*, 1997;126(7):532-538.
14. Altman D. Practical statistics for medical research. London; Chapman & Hall, 1991.
15. Dickersin K, Min YI, Meinert CL. Factors influencing publication of research results. Follow-up of applications submitted to two institutional review boards. *JAMA* 267(3):374-8, 1992.
16. Peto R. Why do we need systematic overviews of randomized trials? Stat Med, 1987;6(3):233-44.
17. Clarke MJ, Stewart LA. Obtaining data from randomised controlled trials: how much do we need for reliable and informative meta-analyses? *BMJ*, 1994; 309(6960): 1007-10.
18. Yusuf S, Wittes J, Probstfield J, Tyroler HA. Analysis and interpretation of treatment effects in subgroups of patients in randomized clinical trials. *JAMA*, 1991; 266 (1):93-98.
19. Fédération Dentaire Internationale (FDI). Principal requirements for controlled clinical trials of caries preventive agents and procedures. Technical report of the commission on oral health, research and epidemiology. *Int Dent J*, 1982;32:292-310.
20. Council on Dental Therapeutics (CDT-ADA). Report of workshop aimed at defining guidelines for caries clinical trials: superiority and equivalency claims for anticaries dentifrices. *JAMA*, 1988; 117:663-5.
21. International Consensus Workshop on Caries Clinical Trials (ICW-CCT) - agreeing where the evidence leads. January 6th-10th 2002. Professors Pitts and Stamm - Co-Chairs. Loch Lomond, 2002.
22. Johnson MF. Comparative efficacy of NaF and SMFP dentifrices in caries prevention: a meta-analytic overview. *Caries Res*, 1993;27:328-36.
23. Helfenstein U, Steiner M. Fluoride varnishes (Duraphat): a meta-analysis. *Community Dent Oral Epidemiol*, 1994, 22:1-5.
24. Stamm JW. Clinical studies of neutral sodium fluoride and sodium monofluorophosphate dentifrices. In: Bowen WH, (eds.). *Relative efficacy of sodium fluoride and sodium monofluorophosphate as anti-caries agents in dentifrices.* London: The Royal Society of Medicine Press Limited; 1995, 43-58.
25. van Rijkom HM, Truin GJ, van't Hof MA. A meta-analysis of clinical studies on the caries-inhibiting effect of fluoride gel treatment. *Caries Res*, 1998;32:83-92.
26. McDonagh MS, Whiting PF, Wilson PM, Sutton AJ, Chestnutt I, Cooper J et al. Systematic review of water fluoridation. *BMJ*, 2000;321:855-9.
27. NHS Centre for Reviews and Dissemination (NHS CRD). A systematic review of public water fluoridation. York: NHS Centre for Reviews and Dissemination, 2000.
28. Bartizek RD, Gerlach RW, Faller RV, Jacobs SA, Bollmer BW, Biesbrock AR. Reduction in dental caries with four concentrations of sodium fluoride in a dentifrice: a meta-analysis evaluation. *J Clin Dent*, 2001;12(3):57-62.
29. Strohmenger L, Brambilla E. The use of fluoride varnishes in the prevention of dental caries: a short review. *Oral Dis*, 2001;7(2):71-80.
30. Marinho VCC, Higgins JPT, Logan S, Sheiham A. Fluoride gels for preventing dental caries in children and adolescents (Cochrane Review). In: The Cochrane Library, Issue 2. Oxford: Update Software; 2002.
31. Marinho VCC, Higgins JPT, Logan S, Sheiham A. Fluoride varnishes for preventing dental caries in children and adolescents (Cochrane Review). In: The Cochrane Library, Issue 2. Oxford: Update Software; 2002.
32. Ammari AB, Bloch-Zupan A, Ashley PF. Systematic review of studies comparing the anti-caries efficacy of children's toothpaste containing 600 ppm of fluoride or less with high fluoride toothpastes with 1,000 ppm or above. *Caries Res*, 2003;37(2):85-92.
33. Marinho VCC, Higgins JPT, Sheiham A, Logan S. Fluoride toothpastes for preventing dental caries in children and adolescents (Cochrane Review). *In:* The Cochrane Library, Issue 1. Oxford: Update Software, 2003.
34. Marinho VCC, Higgins JPT, Sheiham A, Logan S. Fluoride mouthrinses for preventing dental caries in children and adolescents (Cochrane Review). In: The

Cochrane Library, Issue 3. Oxford: Update Software, 2003

35. Stamm JW, Bohannan HM, Graves RC, Disney JA. The efficiency of caries prevention with weekly fluoride mouthrinses. *J Dent Educ*, 1984;48:617-26.
36. Clark DC, Hanley JA, Stamm JW, Weinstein PL. An empirically based system to estimate the effectiveness of caries- preventive agents. A comparison of the effectiveness estimates of APF gels and solutions, and fluoride varnishes. *Caries Res*, 1985;19:83-95.
37. Worthington H, Clarkson J. The evidence base for topical fluorides. *Community Dent Health*, 20:74-76, 2003.
38. Egger M, Smith GD, Phillips AN. Meta-analysis: principles and procedures *BMJ* 1997;315:1533-1537.
39. Jadad AR, Cook DJ, Jones A, et al. Methodology and reports of systematic reviews and meta-analyses: a comparison of Cochrane reviews with articles published in paper-based journals. *JAMA*, 1998;280:278-80.
40. Jadad AR, Moher M, Browman GP, et al. Systematic reviews and meta-analyses on treatment of asthma: critical evaluation. *BMJ*, 2000;320:537-540.
41. Shea B, Dube C, Moher D. Assessing the quality of reports of systematic reviews: the Quorum statement compared to other tools. In: Egger M, Savey Smith G, Altman DG, eds. Systematic reviews in health care: Meta-analysis in context. London: *BMJ*, 2001;122-139.
42. Olsen O, Middleton P, Ezzo J, et al. Quality of Cochrane reviews: assessment of sample from 1998. *BMJ*, 2001;323:829-832.

Influences of social environmental policies on children's health

Healthy public policies have been defined as all general policy developed by governments and public institutions, emphasizing propositions and actions that aim at social change. They highlight a series of activities, reasonably related, with its intentional or non intentional consequences, which can have an impact on the health of the people.[14]

With the definition above, healthy public policies can be seen as part of the health promotion proposals, according to what was defined as the Ottawa Charter, in the Healthy Cities project, [15] and in the Conference of Adelaide about health promotion and healthy public policies, sponsored by the World Health Organization – WHO.[16]

Although based on the same grounds that guide the health promotion paradigm, the healthy public policies can reveal a greater orientation towards public health, social justice, and the structural changes in the society, avoiding the tendency of "victim blaming", which is more probable to arise in strategies that focus on individuals and their lifestyles only.[17-21]

The level of a community healthy public policy implementation can be, potentially, a marker for community factors related to children's health like, for example, recreational equipment and leisure areas, quality and safety at day care centres and schools, condition of the streets, environmental protection, and the kinds of foods that are available. These factors can affect everybody in the community, even though the effects are manifested on the individuals.[22] Moreover, when the concern is aimed to the effects of healthy policies on children, the need is to differentiate between individual effects and the effects of the social context created by the adults.[23]

At this point, it is important to question the relationship of children with the immediate environments of existence and the complexities of their lives, which are determined by structural conditions in which their families live, by the communities that involve them in any way, and the social groups to which they belong. The evidence that the material conditions are associated to health and that people from poor areas have, on average, worse health than those from more prosperous areas seems to be anodyne, after the mass of literature published about the issue. Diez-Roux[24] studied how measures based on areas of poverty and material deprivation are associated with health outcomes. There is evidence of important relationships between, for example, characteristics of neighborhoods and domestic violence; the classification of countries in terms of the Gross National Product and outcomes on fertility; community variables, that modify the effects of maternal education on children's diarrhoea; the kind of health care and immunization on childhood; and the interaction between group variables and individual variables on the transmission of dengue.

Even though there seems to be no direct and simple causal relationship between the level of structural and environmental development of a geo-populational area and the oral health of the people, some studies about traumatic injuries, including dental-facial trauma, in both underdeveloped and emergent countries, seem to contradict such a perception. Trauma in adults, for example, seems to be caused by factors that are external to the house environment, including traffic accidents, urban violence, and occupational risks.[25] However, traumatic accidents with children seem to point out how important are the internal house environment or factors immediately associated to the places where they spend the major part of their daily life, like the day care centres, the schools, or the surroundings of the residential area. This includes the presence of environmental risks of the neighbourhood, the nature and the demographic density of houses and the inappropriate supervision of little children.[25] Traumatic injuries in children have been associated also with sanitation and other physical and environmental characteristics of the residential areas.[26-30]

Another relationship between the level of social environmental development and oral health was found by Moysés,[31] in a study correlating the Human Development Index (HDI) of Brazilian states and the DMF-T index (experience of caries in permanent teeth). This relationship was statistically significant (Graph 9.1). The HDI is, obviously, a potent measure of the social and environmental conditions in which the inhabitants of the states live, reflecting the income, the education, and extremely sensitive indicators like infant mortality. The correlation indicates that the phenomenon of oral-dental health or disease may reflect the same determinant base for the quality of life in general.

Socio-environmental factors frequently are the primary concern and the responsibility of local and state public health institutions. According to the WHO,[32] community social environmental factors that affect oral health include the process of adding fluoride to the water supply, and to toothpastes, policies related to tobacco, alcohol and drugs, preventive oral care subsidized by public and free access, healthy diet, environmental surveillance, and public education for health. More general environmental factors would include the economic context, relative wealth, political participation, social level of tension and violence. These values or conditions are influence the way people see oral health, and whether the services are the responsibility of the individual, of the state or both.

The inclusion of socio-environmental factors as explanations for the oral health of populations has been promising. For example, the classic study of Gratrix and Holloway,[33] in which important inferences were generated about the approach to the social determinants of diseases, correlations were tested between the levels of oral disease and the community characteristics related to health in contrasting neighbourhood areas in relation to affluence. The investigators adopted an ecologic approach, selecting the five schools in which five years old students had the highest experience of dental caries, and another five schools in which children of the same age group had the lowest experience of caries. When the areas were ordered, the communities with a high activity of caries among the children had the lower percentage of babies with normal weight at birth; lower percentages of children with updated immunization, and more children born to separated couples. The communities with a high prevalence of caries also tended to early wean babies, they used

Graph 9.1 Spearman's correlation coefficient for the variables Human Development Index (HDI) and DMF-T, by Brazilian states; Brazil, 1996.

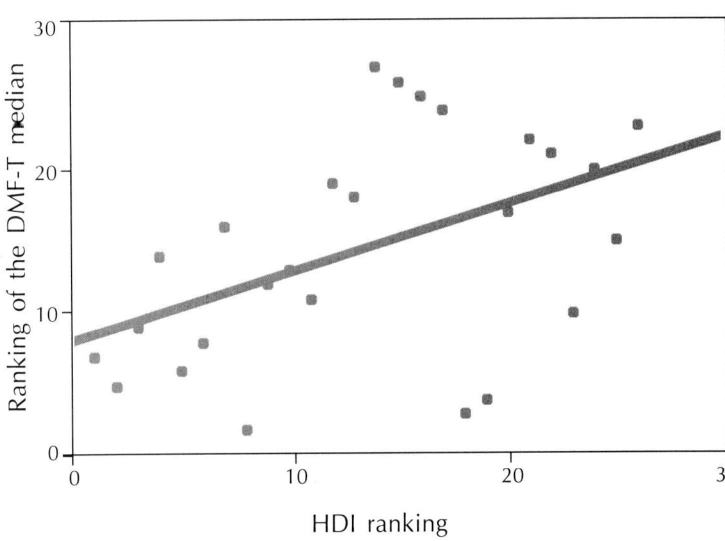

R = 0,47, R2 = 0,22
p = 0,01

prove their own health. The Ottawa Charter for health promotion was drafted in 1984 (WHO 1984) at the first international conference on health promotion. The declaration cites three roles that health care personnel can adopt to promote heath: advocacy, enabling and facilitating.

Advocacy recognises that good health is a major resource for social, economic and personal development and an important dimension of quality of life. Equally it acknowledges the influence that political, economic, social, cultural, environmental, behavioural and biological factors can have on the health of individuals or communities. Advocacy aims to make those conditions favourable to health.

Enabling recognises that people cannot fulfil their fullest health potential unless they are able to take control of the factors which determine their health. Enabling includes providing a supportive environment, access to information, life skills and opportunities for making healthy choices. Health promotion aims to reduce differences in health status between groups and to ensure equal opportunities and resources to enable all people to achieve their fullest health potential.

Mediation recognises that improvements in health can only be achieved through co-ordinated action by governments, health and other social and economic sectors, by non-governmental and voluntary organisations, by local authorities, by industry and the media. Improvements in health involve individuals, families and communities. Professional and social groups and health personnel have a major responsibility to mediate between differing interests in society for the pursuit of health.

Strategies for health promotion

According to the Ottawa charter the pursuit of health follows five strategies. These are building healthy public policy, creating supportive environments, strengthening community action, developing personal skills and reorienting health services.

The charter places the responsibility for health promotion in health services on individuals, community groups, health professionals, health service institutions and governments. All of these must work together to build a health system which contributes to the pursuit of health.

Health services must move beyond responsibility for providing clinical and curative services to promote health. The Charter gives health services an expanded mandate to support the needs of individuals and communities for a healthier life and open channels between the health sector and the broader social, political, economic and environmental components.

This will involve stronger attention to health research as well as professional education and training. This must lead to a change of attitude and organisation of health services which focuses on the total needs of the individual as a whole person.

Therefore reorienting health services implies a shift of service and resource towards health promotion and a sharing of power with other sectors, other disciplines and most importantly with the people themselves.

Oral health as a part of general good health

It is not difficult to interest primary care professionals in promoting oral health within the context of overall good health and well-being. Dental disease can prejudice general health, causing acute pain, distress and lost nights' sleep for the suffering child and for the entire family. As eating becomes uncomfortable chronic pain can affect a child's diet and nutrition.

Dental disease can result in chronic sepsis, producing a bad taste and an unpleasant odour, or in acute sepsis with raised temperature and general malaise.

Acute infection can provoke cellulitis which in extreme cases may present a threat to life.

Dental treatment can be unpleasant, especially for a young child with a limited ability to co-operate and a high treatment need. A general anaesthetic administered to allow extraction of teeth is at best a traumatic experience and at worst is an unnecessary risk to life.

It should always be borne in mind that dental disease is preventable, and that all its consequences and sequelae are therefore avoidable.

The common risk factor approach

A common risk factor approach focuses not on specific illnesses and their prevention but on shared risk factors and their reduction. Risk factors such as nutrition, poor hygiene and smoking will affect levels of dental caries, periodontal disease and oral cancer as well as other cancers, coronary heart disease and stroke, and many other infectious and non-infectious diseases.

The common risk factor approach fits well into a primary care setting, where the interventions that are most likely to be implemented are those which are simple and appropriate. Risk factors are often linked, and someone who is ready to make changes in relation to one factor is likely to be ready to change in relation to another.

By working closely with all members of the primary health care team the prevention of oral disease can take its place in a common risk factor approach. All information the public receive from health professionals should be consistent and correct, thereby maximising the credibility of the message with the target group.

Those with the potential to include oral health education in the advice they give, or to influence oral health through developing policy or creating a supportive environment include doctors, nurses, midwives, dentists and their teams, pharmacists, dietitians or nutritionists, pharmacists and community health workers. If all primary health care professionals work as a team giving scientifically based, consistent advice, and if they reinforce their message through the features of the environment that they provide for their patients and clients, then together they present a formidable alliance in the fight against preventable disease.

Sugar reduction in the context of good overall nutrition

Dental caries can be prevented by restricting the frequency of sugar intake, preferably to mealtimes. Reducing the proportion of fatty foods, and compensating by increasing the proportion of carbohydrate foods such as rice, pasta, bread and potatoes, and increasing the consumption of fresh fruit and vegetables to five portions a day is the diet advocated to reduce the risk of coronary heart disease, cancers and other common diseases.

A diet low in fat and high in complex carbohydrates, fruit and vegetables will naturally lead to a reduction in the intake of sugary foods. Foods such as biscuits, cake and confectionery tend to be high in fat as well as sugars. High sugar foods also displace more nutritious foods from the diet and may lead to obesity. Young people obtain a high proportion of their sugar intake from soft drinks and confectionery. High sugar foods, including sweets and fizzy drinks, contain "empty calories", that is calories with little nutritional value other than their calorie content.

Sugar reduction in the context of good practice in infant feeding

The weaning diet is a particularly important in preparing the pattern for good nutrition throughout life. During weaning a child should be introduced to a range of tastes and textures with the consistency gradually progressing from pureed, through minced or mashed to finely chopped foods.

A healthy weaning diet has as its basis cereals and other carbohydrate foods, fruit and vegetables, gradually incorporating meat, fish, eggs and pulses. Salt and sugar should not be added. (Department of Health 1994). A child who becomes used to a high sugar diet early in life will find it hard to appreciate the range of foods that make up a healthy diet later on in life.

Breast feeding for at least the first four months of life is as desirable in promoting dental health as it is in promoting the overall health and well-being of an infant. Although on-demand feeding after the first teeth have come through may cause dental caries in a few children, on a population basis this is a relatively small problem compared to the effects of sugar-containing drinks in feeding bottles which may be given to non-breast fed children.

Case study 1 – Local infant feeding policy

Many hospitals and community health services in Britain have an infant feeding policy. The aim of this is to standardise the advice that health workers give to parents of young children. The policy will govern the advice given and the content of the health education materials used. It will also provide guidance on wider issues, such as advertising, distribution of samples and other marketing techniques for which baby food manufacturers may seek to use health services premises or personnel, thus implying professional sanction for their product.

The rationale behind an infant feeding policy is to reduce conflicting advice to parents. Parents of young children receive advice from many professional groups including doctors, nurses, community and hospital based midwives and health visitors – who in the United Kingdom monitor development and advise on the health and well-being of 0-4 year olds. Conflicting advice from different health professionals is confusing and sometimes distressing to parents. A local infant feeding policy aims to ensure that all advice is consistent and scientifically based, and that the example set by health professionals and the environment they provide for their patients and clients is congruent with such advice.

The process of developing an infant feeding policy may seem cumbersome and time consuming but is designed to ensure that all professionals involved have a say in the final policy and are therefore willing to conform to it. A working group is established which will normally include a hospital based paediatrician, a community based medical officer, a midwife, a health visitor, a representative from primary care, a nutritionist and a dentist or oral health promoter.

The group will review the existing literature and government guidelines on infant feeding, and will produce the first draft of a policy which is circulated for comments. The process continues until the final draft of a consensus document is produced.

The policy should then be approved by the Boards of the health organisations involved to give it official status. It is then printed and published and distributed to all those in the district who are involved in advising parents on infant feeding. The working group should then plan a launch and a training strategy to ensure that all the professional groups involved are aware of the policy and its contents.

Transferable principles from an infant feeding strategy: importance of early years, multidisciplinary working, consultation, consensus, evidence base, working within government guidelines, dissemination of information supported by training.

Good dental health and primary socialization

Primary health care professionals who have a health education role with the parents of young children have unrivalled opportunities for encouraging the early adoption of routines and behaviours conducive to good dental health for life. Twice daily toothbrushing and a liking for unsweetened foods and drinks are behaviours that if learnt in the first years of life, will continue into adulthood.

The period of primary socialisation, in the first years of life, is the period when habits and routines, many of them health related, are established. The routines of primary socialisation are learnt from those with whom the child has a strong affective relationship: these include family members, particularly the parents. Such behaviours are learnt unquestioningly as a taken-for-granted reality. Habits and routines are particularly important in health related behaviour, because they are dependable. Because they require no thought or intention they are more reliable than decision-based behaviours which readily break down under stress.

Other risk factors

Good oral hygiene is a natural part of good hygiene and grooming. Those who have no cleanliness or grooming routine tend to have poor oral hygiene. Toothbrushing is most effectively learnt in the first years of life, through the process of primary socialisation, from other family members. It will usually be learnt as part of a routine which includes washing and bathing or showering. Good oral hygiene is valued by most people because it makes their mouth and teeth look good, smell nice, and feel pleasant. The social aspects of good oral hygiene are probably the greatest motivators for tooth brushing.

Thorough twice-daily tooth brushing with fluoride toothpaste prevents dental disease in two ways. Brushing removes from the gum margin the plaque or layer of germs that causes gingivitis (swollen and bleeding gums) and periodontal disease (loss of the tooth's attachment to the jawbone). Tooth brushing is also an effective method of applying fluoride to the teeth. If toothpaste is applied at least once, and preferable twice a day, it strengthens the enamel of the teeth and will reduce tooth decay. Tooth brushing is an acceptable way of applying fluoride to the teeth because it enjoys great social support.

Many young people suffer from trauma to their front teeth while playing or taking part in sport. This can be reduced by efforts to make the environment safer, as well as by promoting the use of gum shields in contact sports.

Smoking is the most important risk factor for lung and other cancers, for coronary heart disease, stroke, and other circulatory diseases. In adults it also predisposes to periodontal disease, and can mask the symptoms by suppressing bleeding while the disease progresses. Along with alcohol consumption is an important risk factor for oral cancer. Therefore primary prevention of smoking, that is discouraging children from taking up the habit, is a part of promoting long-term oral health.

Multidisciplinary approach

Multidisciplinary working is implicit in the common risk factor approach. The fact that particular risk factors are common to a number of different health problems will help to bring different groups together to reduce threats to health. Multidisciplinary working is a fundamental principle of health promotion, as many disciplines and sectors can influence the determinants of health. What makes multidisciplinary work a challenge to many professionals is that it requires a shared agenda, negotiation of priorities and stepping outside of traditional ways of working.

Promoting oral health through a multidisciplinary approach requires an analysis of which professions, groups, disciplines or sectors can affect the determinants of oral health, through advocacy, enabling or mediation. Some will build oral health into policies, others can create supportive environments or make healthy choices easier choices for the target groups. Some will build individuals' knowledge and skills, while others will be involved in supporting the development of communities.

Raising the profile of oral health with primary health care professionals

The first step to involving different primary care professionals in promoting oral health is to convince them that oral disease threatens the health and well-being of their clients or patients. They may have seen this themselves at first hand, and have witnessed the infection, pain, loss of function, loss of aesthetics or anxiety that dental disease or its treatment can generate.

Training is the key to involving different professional groups in oral health promotion and will be discussed in more detail in subsequent sections. Meetings with key individuals, speaking at meetings and participatory training can all raise the profile of oral health.

The media can also be useful in promoting the importance and relevance of good oral health with primary health care professionals and with others who can influence the determinants of oral health. The media may include national or local newspapers, local or national radio or television, the web, professional journals, magazines or newsletters. A constant low key issue of information through these channels builds and maintains awareness. Locally relevant information is particularly interesting to local primary health care professionals.

Planning an intervention with primary health care professionals

The next stage involves information gathering. What is needed first is an overview of the pressures, priorities and preoccupations of the particular professional group. It may be a particularly opportune moment to work with them as their focus shifts to adopting a public health role or promoting good nutrition. Or the time may not be right, for example if they are feeling threatened by organisational change.

The most important thing to do when planning an intervention with a group of primary care professionals is to listen well. It may be valuable to talk to several representatives of the profession. Those in a position of power and influence or who act as representatives of the profession will be key allies. But it is those who work on the frontline with the general public on a day-to-day basis that will actually have to implement any initiative. Their very realistic and practical perspective will be another important contribution to the planning process.

These representatives of the profession will be able to identify how the group can promote oral health as part of their everyday work. This will depend on whether health education and promotion is an integral part of what they do, what are their priorities, how pressured is their workload and the degree of autonomy they have in their work.

If the programme is to take place on at a national or regional level the appropriate professional organisation should be involved. If it is a local programme or campaign then the support of managers is essential and that of local representatives of the professional organisation is very helpful.

The training and resource needs of the group should be assessed. These will be discussed in more detail later in the chapter. It is wise to pilot any new programme with a few members of the discipline who are enthusiastic and well motivated about dental health. As the programme is implemented it will need to be carefully monitored to see if it is functioning as intended. If it is not then the reasons for this should be assessed and any necessary adjustments should be made and improvements built in to the process.

These activities may be co-ordinated by an individual or a small team. Larger scale projects may be overseen by a working party which will gather together the necessary interests and expertise.

Case study 2– The North West Dental Health Education Campaign: working with health visitors and dentists

In 1988 the British Government published a policy document on promoting better health which included a section advocating initiatives to promote dental awareness and regular attendance at the dentist, especially among the young and those in deprived area. Funding was made available for this purpose through the Government's then lead agency in promoting health, the Health Education Authority.

The North West Region of England (Greater Manchester and Lancashire) was selected as its population suffered poor general health and poor dental health, with caries levels in children the highest in the English regions. The region suffers from high levels of social deprivation, a high proportion of the population are classified among the lower social classes and among these are a high proportion of ethnic minorities and of very young mothers.

The region also enjoyed close co-operation between then Regional Health Authority, the University Dental School and the Community Dental Service, and had strong traditions of health education, health promotion and health services research.

The aim of the campaign was to improve the dental health of young people in the North Western Region by focussing on young parents and their children, on health professionals in a position to contact and influence this target group and on the availability of dental services in deprived areas.

A key objective was to increase the involvement of appropriate professionals including general dental practitioners, nurses, health visitors, nursery nurses and pharmacists. One of the main strands of the programme was a campaign aimed at young mothers and their children working through appropriate professionals.

Health visitors were identified as the key group in the campaign. Health visitors are specially trained nurses whose role is to monitor and promote the healthy development of young children. They do this through a combination of visiting parents at home, running sessions in local clinics and through public health work. They are employed by the local community health services but work closely with general medical practices.

The first step in the campaign was to undertake a baseline survey of the dental health knowledge, beliefs and behaviours of health visitors in the region. Meanwhile a regional steering group was established which included specialists in dental public health, health visitors, a health visitor manager, a community nutritionist, a health promotion specialist and a press officer. The combination was invaluable. It provided wide based expertise, allowing the preparation of relevant and sound materials and resources and their dissemination, and of training which was relevant and appropriate to the health visitors' needs. Importantly too it improved communication with the various professions represented and encouraged their involvement. The steering group met monthly from October 1988 to April 1989 and determined precisely the target group, planned the workshops and decided what materials would be used in the campaign.

Resources were produced for the health visitors to use. These included posters for clinics, leaflets for the public, a manual for health visitors on promoting oral health, a copy of the policy document "The scientific basis of dental health education", and a strip of pictures for the health visitors to use with their clients showing healthy teeth, feeding bottle caries, clean teeth and plaque covered teeth.

Ten workshops were held in five venues at the beginning of January 1989, in order to brief the health visitors before the launch of an advertising campaign which aimed to discourage mothers from giving sugary foods and drinks to their children. The survey of health visitors had already shown that they knew a lot about dental health, so the workshops needed not so much to pass on information as to seek health visitors' support in giving advice to the target group.
The aims of the workshops were:

1. To provide health visitors with an update on the aetiology and prevention of dental disease, particularly in young children.
2. To provide an opportunity for health visitors to discuss how they might promote dental health in small children as part of their existing role as health promoters
3. To explain the accompanying advertising campaign.

The workshops took the form of short presentations by expert speakers, followed by working groups and a plenary discussion. Attendance at the workshops was high, and their evaluation of the event was good. The workshops generated valuable ideas about what advice to give, when and to whom. These are presented here as they offer a good example of how a professional group can themselves suggest how oral health fits in to their everyday work.

1. What advice?

- Antenatal advice to breast feed.
- Accept that some sugar will be given and encourage parents to limit its frequency and avoid bedtimes.
- Encourage regular family eating patterns.
- Introduce a feeding cup instead of a bottle as early as possible.
- Give parents positive suggestions about suitable foods to give.
- Try and get mothers to realise that a good baby is not one that is always sleeping.
- Get mothers to feel positive about their own health.

2. When to give advice?

- Dental health education can be incorporated into routine work in the first year of life establishing healthy habits and routines, at parentcraft classes, teething consultations, baby clinics and hearing tests.

3. Who to give advice to?

- To teenagers to reduce their own sugar consumption and taste for sweet foods before they themselves become parents; to parents, and to the whole extended family

4. Resources

- Health visitors asked for leaflets, posters, lists of dentists, pictures of decayed teeth to show to their clients, videos, tooth brushes and tooth paste.

5. Inter-sectoral collaboration
   Health visitors asked for a dental input into their training and that of midwives. They also considered that they themselves could make a valuable input into the training of dentists. They recommended that doctors should get training in oral health too and should be encouraged to prescribe sugar-free medicines. They thought it important that each district should have an infant feeding and weaning policy and in-service training to ensure its implementation. They affirmed that all health professionals have a role in promoting dental health and should give consistent advice.

Making healthy choices easier choices

Setting a good example, by not selling sugary drinks on health service premises, by not giving sweets as rewards after inoculations, by not distributing commercial baby food samples packs on health service premises which contain sugared foods and drinks. Health visitors could also, as individuals and as a professional group, act as advocates for the manufacture of sugar-free baby foods and drinks

Seminars were also held for general dental practitioners. Dentists were seen as an important source of advice for mothers about caring for their children's teeth. Health visitors were recommending to mothers that they took their young children along to the dentist so that it was important that dentists put the children on their lists of patients and advised the parents about how to prevent dental disease.

Transferable principles from the North West Dental Health Education campaign: early years work, multidisciplinary working, assessing training need and need for resources, encouraging professionals to produce their own ideas for their role in promoting oral health, training seminars, production of suitable resources.

Team working

A team is a group of people who work together to achieve a common goal. This involves a number of people combining their different skills so that the best use is made of each person's individual abilities, at the same time helping the team to achieve its tasks.

In primary health care team working is seen as a way of delivering co-ordinated care, widening skills and improving the quality of the patient's experience. Effective team work is achieved through careful planning, development and good communication.

A team is a group of people who have come together for a common purpose. They are characterised by a basic interdependence, by their need to communicate and work together to achieve their purpose and by each of them having a defined role within the team to help achieve the team goal. Working as a team leads to more effective working, more efficient use of staff and better staff motivation.

Fundamental requisites of an ideally functioning team are:

- The team must have a meaningful, clearly defined task
- There should be clear team objectives
- Its members should have unique and meaningful tasks
- Performance of individual members should be assessed and they should receive feedback
- There should be regular feedback on the team's successes
- The team should be reflexive, that is able to change
- All members of the team should be fully participative

Team working is very important to promoting the oral health of the young child. Most health care settings are made up of teams, usually led by a health professional such as a doctor, pharmacist or dentist. Each member of the team can have a role in promoting oral health. What is important is that a policy is agreed and that everyone in the team is clear about what their own and other team members' responsibilities are in relation to promoting oral health.

General dental practitioners can use a teamwork approach to promoting the dental health of children. This will help them work more effectively, ensuring that appropriate and timely advice is given to the patients who need it. The practice will function more efficiently, because some oral health education tasks will be delegated to auxiliary staff rather than carried out by the dentist. This approach also improves morale within the practice as dental nurses and receptionists are often keen to widen their role, use their abilities and develop their skills.

First the task must be defined, and each dental team member's contribution agreed and communicated. Staff meetings form ideal opportunities for this. Agreement will be reached on which patients should receive health education advice, what advice they should receive, where, when and from whom. Then the role of each individual staff member should be defined. For example the dentist will be responsible for including prevention in the treatment plan, and may review the patient's progress at subsequent visits. A dental nurse may be trained to carry out toothbrush instruction or to assess and advise on the child's sugar intake. The receptionist might be in charge of health education materials and making sure these are displayed or given to appropriate patients.

Regular meetings and reviews should be held to check that the agreed system is working well, enabling individual team members to reflect on their own performance and to suggest changes and improvements to the system. The dentist can use this as an opportunity to give feedback to staff about individual and collective successes in improving patients' oral health related behaviours.

Teamwork also forms the basis of multidisciplinary projects or programmes to improve the oral health of children.

Case study 3; The oral health promoting medical practice

The oral health promoting practice scheme operates in two districts with poor dental health in the North West of England. It is an idea that was originally suggested by a primary care development nurse and it has proved popular and successful with primary health care teams.

The aim of the scheme is to promote oral health through the primary health care team. The first stage is to raise team members' awareness of the poor state of oral health in the area and how dental disease affects general health and well-being. This is carried out through work with individual team members and through presentations at team meetings. The team is asked to make a commitment to promoting oral health and to produce a very brief written statement to that effect.

The commitment includes an agreement to fulfil defined criteria. These are: to prescribe sugar-free medicines; to not use sweets as rewards (instead badges and stickers are provided for children for after vaccinations and other unpleasant procedures); not to promote sugar-containing baby foods and drinks, for example by adverts or samples; to promote dental registration and to display dental health education materials supplied by the dental health promotion team.

Each team member has a specific role. For example doctors prescribe sugar-free medicines, practice nurses are responsible for rewards and for dental health education materials, community midwives control marketing of baby products in the practice and receptionists check that new patients are regular dental attenders.

The practice is formally presented with a certificate recognising their achievement, and the local press informed of the award. Individual members of the team are revisited regularly to keep them supplied with resources and to get feedback on the scheme. The scheme is constantly developing and evolving on the basis of suggestions made by primary care team members.

Every couple of years the practice team is revisited to give formal thanks and acknowledge their contribution to improving dental health. Almost all the practices in the area participate in the scheme. Since the scheme began there has been an increase in the proportion of sugar-free prescriptions written.

A parallel scheme operates with pharmacy teams. This is discussed below.

Transferable principles: team working, common defined goal, each team member with clearly defined role, feedback and on-going development.

A settings approach

The oral health promoting medical practice scheme uses the principles of a settings approach. The implicit message is that oral health is taken seriously. A settings approach looks at systems within an organization or institution and treats the daily activities there in a holistic way. It uses both health promotion as a way of creating a healthy environment and health education as a means of enabling people to achieve lifestyles conducive to health.

The theory behind a settings approach is that health promotion becomes an integral part of the general climate of the organisation or institution – part of the way it is managed and part of the extended care provided for its clients. This includes the social and physical environment. The settings approach involves primary care professionals in the roles of enabling, mediating and advocacy.

Such an approach to oral health promotion within a setting leads to its staff assessing their activities for their potential effect on oral health. Whenever possible the activity is used as an opportunity to promote oral health, for example dietary advice will include sugar reduction. It is also used to ensure that any potential damage to oral health is minimised, for example by substituting a sugar-free medicine for one which contains sugar.

Case study 4 – The oral health promoting pharmacy

The oral health promoting pharmacy scheme recognises that customers are not just influenced by the advice they receive but also by the environment of the pharmacy itself. In the United Kingdom pharmacists dispense prescriptions and sell over-the-counter medicines as well as a wide range of health related products, baby foods, cosmetic and other products.

The oral health promoting pharmacy scheme complements the oral health promoting medical practice scheme described above. Oral health promoting pharmacies:

1 Do not sell confectionery.
2. Prominently display and recommend sugar-free alternatives including over-the-counter medicines, drinks and baby products.
3. Staff take part in a training session on oral health problems, prevention and products.
4. Dental health posters and leaflets are displayed and dispensed.

It is interesting to reflect on the limitations of this scheme in practice. Unlike medical practices, pharmacies in the

United Kingdom combine the role of primary care setting with that of profit driven businesses. (The same applies to general dental practices in the UK.) Therefore the extent to which pharmacy staff – who furthermore are often employees of a multiple chain – can adhere to the standards of the scheme is limited.

For example the sale of confectionery is an important income generator and so staff may be unable to discontinue the practice. However the scheme aims to encourage improvements in practice. Therefore a different level of award is available to recognise the efforts of pharmacy teams who fulfil the other criteria, but are able to do no more than restrict the sale of confectionery to away from the medicines counter.

Training the primary health care team in promoting oral health

Training is pivotal to any strategy to promote oral health through the primary health care team. All primary care staff who will be involved in promoting oral health will need training and periodic updating.

Training need

The first step is to identify the training needs of the group. Their needs will be determined by the extent to which health promotion (enabling, advocacy or mediating) forms a part of their work, by how great a priority oral health promotion is for them, by how much time they have available for training, their baseline knowledge, the needs of their patients or clients and their own interest in the subject. Training needs can be assessed by means of discussion with the primary health care professionals themselves, or with their managers or representatives.

Promoting the uptake of training

Most primary health care professionals are busy people. Health promotion is often a low priority, and oral health promotion even less important. Therefore it is essential that training is made as convenient as possible and that it should be absolutely relevant to their needs (see Case Studies).

The training might be made convenient for primary health care workers by holding it as part of a meeting which they would attend anyway, or by holding it in their work place or at a time that they choose. Planning the training with advice from the group themselves, and then evaluating it formally and informally will ensure that the training is relevant to the group and constantly evolves to meet their changing needs.

A particular campaign may demand a programme of one-off training sessions. Often however training will take the form of regular updates, each session building on the last, gradually developing the group's expertise in and commitment to oral health. If, as a part of the training, the group or professionals are provided with good quality resources tailored to meet their own needs and those of their client group, this will provide a further incentive for taking part in the training.

Oral health promotion should ideally form a part of the training of medical students, student nurses and midwives, dental and pharmacy students and any other specialists in community health or medicine.

Content of training

The content of the training will be determined by the training needs analysis. Dental and non-dental staff will probably need an update on the scientific basis of dental health education, and on the particular oral health messages that relate to the needs of their client group. Infants, younger and older children and adolescents will all have different needs at their different stages of development.

The content will include relevant aspects of the causes and prevention of tooth decay, gum disease, dental trauma and oral cancer. Participants may be asked to reflect on their opportunities for including oral health in their work, whether by enabling, mediation or advocacy.

Primary health care professionals respond to information which is locally relevant. This may describe the main oral health problems in the locality, compare the local and national picture and provide information on which groups within the local child population are most at risk from dental disease.

Oral health promotion for the primary dental care team

Although the dental team have a highly developed knowledge and understanding of the treatment of dental disease, they may need updating on health education messages and techniques. Models of individual behaviour change, dealt with later in the chapter, may help them to structure their advice and give it at an opportune time. Training for the dental team may also include the development of communication skills and a team approach.

Their training needs may also include a consideration of oral health in the wider context of nutrition and hygiene. The dental team has been trained to focus on individual health, rather than the wider determinants that affect the health and oral health of communities. A public health perspective can help them to understand why it is that their patients do not always follow their advice, and some of the social and economic factors that influence their patients' behaviour.

Methods of training for primary health care professionals

Primary health care professionals have a great deal of background knowledge and personal and professional experience. Training can give participants the chance to reflect on this experience, structure it and use it to identify opportunities for oral health promotion. On the basis of this they can then identify and fill any gaps in relevant knowledge.

Training for adults is essentially participative and interactive. If training is to be provided for large numbers they may be split into groups to define problems and generate solutions. For example primary health care professionals may be asked to discuss the effect that dental health problems have on their clients' general health and well being, and what they can do to improve their clients' oral health. Feedback, questions and discussion are an important part of the process.

With a smaller group training may be much more informal and less obviously structured, although the underlying objectives would be similar. Participation can be encouraged in a much more natural manner.

Training should be evaluated. Formal methods include semi-structured questionnaires. Informal evaluation may take the form of a discussion of what aspects of the training the participants found most useful.

Case study 5– the Baby Welcome scheme

The Baby Welcome scheme was developed in two districts in the North West of England in response to a fundamental contradiction. Dental health in the area was extremely poor despite the very high percentage of 0-2 year olds who had attended the dentist.

Anecdotal evidence was that although